THE MINISTRY OF BODIES

SEAMUS O'MAHONY

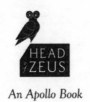

An Apollo Book

An Apollo book
First published in the UK in 2021
by Head of Zeus Ltd

Copyright © Seamus O'Mahony, 2021

9 7 5 3 2 4 6 8

A catalogue record for this book is available from
the British Library.

ISBN (HB): 9781838931926
ISBN (XTPB): 9781800244221
ISBN (E): 9781838931940

Printed and bound in Great Britain by
CPI Group (UK) Ltd, Croydon CRO 4YY

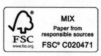

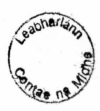

Head of Zeus Ltd
5–8 Hardwick Street
London ECIR 4RG
WWW.HEADOFZEUS.COM

THE MINISTRY
OF BODIES

SEAMUS O'MAHONY spent many years working for the National Health Service in Britain. He now lives in his native Cork, in the south of Ireland. His acclaimed first book, *The Way We Die Now*, was published in 2016, and won a British Medical Association Book Award in 2017. *Can Medicine Be Cured?* (2019), his sharp and witty critique of the medical profession, has so far been translated into three languages.

Contents

To Karen, James and Helena

Introduction

This book is based on notes – not really a diary – I kept over the last eight months of my career as a doctor. I decided to retire some months after I had started writing these notes. I left just before The Thing; the world I have written about now seems remote, a time of lost content. The 'ministry' is a large Irish teaching hospital where I worked for many years. The events and people I have written about are 'set' in a variety of locations, including the emergency department, the general wards, the intensive care unit, the outpatient clinic and the endoscopy unit.

I have quoted numerous emails, as they give a flavour not only of the ministry's institutional culture but also of the foolishness of contemporary health care. These emails came from a variety of sources, including hospital management, the regional health service headquarters, the Dublin-based head office of the health service, the local medical school, and – most numerous – individuals at the ministry who felt their message merited the attention of 'all users'. Every day seemed to be consecrated to raising my awareness of a different disease, disability, field of research or human virtue. These communications were so numerous that I could easily have spent my days reading them instead of seeing patients.

Writing about 'real' patients is difficult. I plead the usual weaselly disclaimer: every 'patient' described in this book is a composite of several people I have known over nearly four decades. I have altered their personal details so comprehensively that no individual can be identified.

Writing about other doctors is even more difficult. Those I admired I have presented largely unaltered. The others, like the patients, are amalgams of many doctors I have worked with over the years in hospitals in three countries. If you think you recognise yourself in these pages, and do not like what you read, tell yourself that this is a novel, and any similarity to actual persons, as they say, is purely coincidental.

The ministry and me

I have put more thought into the purchase of certain suits than into my choice of career. I had no pressing sense of philanthropy or vocation. Nowadays, when all aspiring entrants to medical school routinely and formulaically declare their altruism, this is a vaguely shocking admission. Despite these feverish protestations, young people still become doctors for the same reasons as previous generations: status and a good living. There is a lot of humbug: medical school applicants rarely put down social work or nursing as their second choice of course.

Medicine, more than most careers, colonises the lives of its practitioners. I long ago accepted that 'doctor' was my defining role, the first word to come to mind when my name was mentioned, or even when I thought of myself, in some abstract, detached way. I have little doubt – with the benefit of forty years of hindsight – that my personality would have been better suited to a more contemplative life. But circumstances decreed that I should spend four decades pursuing a profession for which, when I started training for it as a teenager,

I had no outstanding aptitude or suitability, apart from a knack of doing well in examinations.

⁓

The ministry and I grew up together. It was built on a large brownfield site in Wilton, in the western suburbs of Cork, near – appropriately – the great necropolis of St Finbarr. I lived nearby and knew this site, known then as the African Missions fields, because it was adjacent to the church and apostolic college of St Joseph, where the Society of African Missions (*Societas Missionum ad Afros* or SMA) once trained young men to be missionary priests in Africa. As a boy, I was always wary of crossing this wasteland, which was patrolled by the Rogers, feral boys from Roger Casement Park, a local council estate. I do not suppose any of the Rogers made the short journey to St Joseph's college to study for the priesthood.

I started medical school in October 1978; the ministry opened the next month. It was the main teaching hospital for the medical school, and the wonder of the age. On the day the ministry opened – 30 November 1978 – the front page of *The Cork Examiner* proudly proclaimed: 'After 40 years, the hospital doors open at... The Wilton Hilton!' 'De Paper'* rather lost the run of itself: 'The first patients may be forgiven if they feel they have been taken not into a hospital, but some wonderful time tunnel to the automated future that their

---

* *The Cork Examiner* (now the *Irish Examiner*) is affectionately known in Cork as 'de paper'. The 'de' is a self-referential joke about the prominent dentalisation of words such as 'this', 'that' and 'the' when spoken with a pronounced Cork accent.

great-grandchildren might know. The 40-year wait was un-questionably worthwhile for today's patient; they will find an environment that would embarrass any top class hotel and their ailment will be analysed and treated by machines that make *Star Wars* look like a scrapyard.'

The architect who designed the ministry was a Yorkshire-man called Richard De'Ath. He specialised in hospitals and universities; his buildings were described by the Royal Institute of British Architects as 'complex' and 'very successful in their function as well as very satisfying visually'. The ministry hasn't aged well; it now looks like a neglected apartment block in some remote post-Soviet city. The Russians have a name for it: 'Khrushchyovka' – low-cost concrete-panelled or brick buildings thrown up during the Khrushchev era. The doctors and nurses who moved from the old hospital (which was built as a workhouse in 1840) to the ministry were so proud, so hopeful, but as the years passed it became, like all such institutions, the repository for problems it was never designed to accommodate, much less solve.

The main 1978 ministry building is a six-storey block with red-brick walls; several squat one- and two-storey flat-roofed ancillary buildings extend from it like crab claws. The red walls are studded with white balconies leading from the wards: did Mr De'Ath anticipate that sitting out in the warm Cork sunshine would contribute to the patients' recovery? Fresh air and sunshine ('heliotherapy') were, after all, the cornerstone of 'treatment' for tuberculosis in the days before antibiotics. Free access to the balconies lasted for a few short years only; I witnessed in 1984 the grisly fall to earth of a man with *delirium tremens* who had flung himself from a top-floor balcony. The doors leading to them may have been shut, but the white balconies remain, a tribute to Mr De'Ath's quixotic expectation of Irish weather. (Perhaps I'm reading too much into the balconies; they may have been added simply for the convenience of the window cleaners.)

There were two wards on each floor; in a break with tradition, the wards were not named after saints, but instead were simply given the number of the floor, followed by either 'a' or 'b'. My 'home' ward was 1b. Each ward had thirty-four beds, comprised of a four-bed 'observation' unit (for the sickest patients), four six-bed rooms, four single rooms (for the infected and the dying) and one double room. The only sop to privacy in the shared rooms – where most of the patients were accommodated – was the flimsy brown-green patterned curtains. The floors were of linoleum and the low ceilings were covered in cheap white styrofoam tiles. It was rumoured that a great deal of asbestos was later removed. When the ministry was young, the walls were painted in various pale shades of green, brown and yellow; over the years, they all became off-white.

The windswept African Missions fields covered many acres, which allowed for the gradual expansion of the ministry into a campus. Little happened during the economically arid 1980s and '90s; the ministry just survived. In 2007 the new maternity hospital opened, connected by a link corridor to the main hospital. This new hospital united on one site maternity services from three old hospitals in the city, one of them private. (Huge medical negligence awards had made private obstetrics unviable, because the obstetricians could no longer afford professional indemnity insurance.) With its modern triangular design, the maternity hospital made the original ministry building look a bit dowdy. Seen from the road, this new wing has a vaguely nautical appearance, with its curved walls and narrow windows. I have always been dubious about the notion that architecture affects behaviour, but when I witnessed the swagger of the obstetricians who came to work at the new hospital, I had to reconsider.

The next development was the cardiac renal centre, completed in 2010,* in the middle of a deep recession: the funding had been signed off before this collapse. Built on five levels, this new wing almost entirely obscures the tatty 1978 building. As its name suggests, it houses services devoted to the care of patients with heart and kidney problems; it is a testament to the political skills of the doctors specialising in these diseases and a permanent monument to the sad reality that some diseases are indeed *better* than others. The centre has a vast, light-filled central atrium, with Pompidou Centre-like glass elevators. At ground level in this atrium, there is a space for concerts (with a grand piano) and a branch of the punningly named café, the 'coffee dock', where the cardiac and renal doctors, wearing modish blue 'scrubs' tops, drink cappuccinos and, no doubt, contemplate their good fortune to be working in such a congenial environment. Even though the main ministry building can be reached via a short corridor, these doctors leave their beautiful edifice under duress only. They regard the old hospital as a *bothán*, a peasant's cabin, fit only for peasants.

The most recent development in the ministry is the radiation oncology Glandore Centre, an imposing building with

* The centre was formally opened by Irish prime minister Brian Cowen in 2011, one of his last official engagements as Taoiseach. He had presided over the catastrophic collapse of the Irish economy. At the time of this formal opening, Cowen was a disgraced, haunted man; he was jeered on arrival by a crowd of 'republicans'.

shiny grey walls at the rear of the old hospital. Its stern exterior seems to say: 'Cancer is a serious business'. There is an unquestioned consensus that cancer is better than all other diseases – even those of the heart and kidneys.

I worked at the hospital, in various capacities, over three spells, for twenty-two years. After graduating in 1983, I trained there for four years. Like most Irish doctors in those days, I emigrated, spending fourteen years in the British National Health Service (NHS). I came back to Cork in 2001. We have disappointed each other, the ministry and me, as we grew from the breezy optimism of youth into crabbed middle age.

The ministry was an oasis of kindness and comfort. It was also a place of chaos and conflict, of institutional cruelty. In *Nothing to Be Frightened of*, Julian Barnes wrote about his year teaching at a Catholic school in Brittany: 'The priests I lived among surprised me by being as humanly various as civilians.' So too with those we now call 'healthcare workers'. Those who have nothing to do with hospitals assume that the people who work in them are saintly and, since the pandemic, 'heroes'. They may be surprised to learn that they are no better, and no worse, than themselves.

'Only God can judge me'

For fourteen years I was one of just two consultants in the gastroenterology department; we eventually – slightly too late for *me* – grew to four. We shared inpatient duties and on-call, spending half our time 'on' for the wards. When 'off' the wards, we did our 'elective' outpatient clinics and endoscopy lists. When 'on' the wards, we did *everything*: on-call, ward rounds, outpatient clinics, endoscopy. Our department sometimes had over sixty inpatients, looked after by two of the four consultants, who rotated this duty. By the time I reached my late fifties, this workload had become intolerable.

The inpatients were a mixture of general medical patients and people with what were deemed to be specifically gastroenterology ('gastro') problems.* The general medical patients came under our care through what was called acute 'take': when on 'take', or call, for general medicine, we took those

---

* Gastroenterology deals with diseases of the stomach, intestine, liver, biliary system and pancreas. Liver disease – traditionally a branch of gastroenterology – is now so prevalent that, in many large hospitals, there are units and doctors ('hepatologists') who deal solely with this.

patients whose problem – usually *problems* – made them unsuitable for admission under specialist departments such as cardiology and neurology, who took only those patients whose problem was deemed to be specifically within their remit. Most 'medical' (as opposed to 'surgical') patients were frail elderly people who were allocated to the physician or department on 'take'. The byzantine rules governing medical 'take' had been laid down forty years before, when the ministry opened, and were seen to be as unalterable as the tablets of stone, immune to the dramatic changes in medicine and demography over those four decades.

Roughly half the inpatients under the care of our department were general medical, and half were 'gastro'. Most of the 'gastro' patients had alcoholic liver disease. When I started in the 1980s, liver cirrhosis was relatively uncommon in Ireland. Despite the lazy racial stereotype, the Irish in those days were, *per capita*, modest consumers of alcohol compared to other Europeans, such as the French and the Spanish. Many people of my parents' generation were teetotal, often for religious reasons, being members of the Catholic Pioneer Total Abstinence Association. By the 1990s and 2000s, Ireland's alcohol consumption had risen sharply, leading to an epidemic of chronic liver disease. This epidemic also took hold in Britain. I spent much of my consultant career at the ministry caring for the victims of this epidemic.

When a colleague handed over ward duties to me, the short summary of a patient given the day before in the 'handover' didn't always conform to what I saw on the ward round. 'Oh, don't worry about Mr Murphy,' they would say, 'he'll probably be gone by tomorrow', or 'he's waiting placement in a nursing home', or 'there's nothing more to be done; he's dying'. Then I did the ward round, and found Mr Murphy's family gathered around the bed, wanting to know why he was still waiting for a CT scan, and why hadn't he been referred to a geriatrician, and could somebody *please* tell us what's happening with Dad?

The ward round was once the central ritual of life in the ministry, where all important decisions on patient care were made. The round had designated days and starting times, and the team of doctors (consultant and juniors) were joined by the most senior nurse. The *ward* round was just that: it started and finished on *one* ward. When the ministry was new, there were even *teaching* rounds. Then, all the doctors wore white coats and the nurses wore white uniforms. There was an office in the basement laundry where clean starched white coats could be picked up on Monday mornings. The many generous pockets in these coats could easily accommodate a stethoscope, bleep, a copy of the *British National Formulary* (for guidance on drugs), several pens, an ophthalmoscope, a packet of cigarettes and a lighter. Now, white coats have been banned on the grounds that they pose an infection risk; two refusenik consultants continued to wear them. The junior doctors wear either theatre 'scrubs' or 'smart casual' attire, and *never* a tie. The senior nurses wear a striped blue and white top with blue pants, while the junior nurses are attired in white. The 'allied health professionals' – physiotherapists, pharmacists and speech and language therapists – are easily identifiable by the colour of their tops, being, respectively, white, green and red.

Four decades on, the ward round continued, but bore little resemblance to the choreographed event of my youth. Over several hours and multiple locations, the 'team' often got broken up. One of them might stay behind on a ward to write up medications or order X-rays; nurses often phoned the juniors after we had left the ward to find out what we had decided. Meanwhile, the wards we had not yet visited would call, wondering when we would arrive; smartphones provided endless opportunities for interruption. I generally began the round with a team of three or four (rising in seniority from intern to senior house officer [SHO] to registrar), but this usually dwindled to one or two as they were called away to attend to something else more pressing. Outside my home ward, the nurses were less attentive and the charts more difficult to find. Rival and competing conversations often took place at a patient's bedside. While I was trying to take a history from an old, deaf, mildly demented patient, a physiotherapist might be next to me, discussing *another* patient with my senior house officer. Record-keeping was ad hoc and haphazard, with the juniors writing in the notes *their* rough interpretation of *my* assessments and plans. These synopses were sometimes wildly incorrect.

But the main problem with rounds was decision-making. A round could not last longer than three hours; the team needed enough time to act on the agreed plan. Assuming thirty patients over three hours (I had very often seen more than fifty), that gave an average of six minutes per patient. For many, no major decision was required: they were working their way through treatment and investigations already planned and agreed; other patients were awaiting 'placement' in nursing homes. Six minutes was enough. For many others, however, six minutes was spectacularly inadequate: they might be new to me; they might not be responding to treatment; they – or their relatives – might require personal time with me; one or two might be acutely sick and in need of urgent attention.

Important decisions, therefore, had to be made quickly, very often without all the necessary information. On an average round, there were perhaps ten to fifteen such decisions to be made. More than once, I had committed errors under this intense pressure. After a major blunder, I knew I had to find a way of managing this. I developed an acute awareness of uncertainty and my own limitations. If I felt unsure, I told the patient. I explained that I couldn't make that decision right now, that I needed to think about their problem, or take advice. I felt no shame in saying this.

When I took over ward duties this morning, I had only twelve patients to see, but it took over two hours: I didn't know them, and they were scattered all over the hospital. Most acutely admitted patients came in through the emergency department, where they were accommodated on trolleys for hours or days, and then sent to wherever a bed could be found 'up the house'. I struggled with some and hoped that the registrar and senior house officer were doing a vague approximation of the right thing.

Sharon, a patient whom I had encountered on previous periods of ward duty, was more complex than most. She had many problems; a solution to these would be unlikely, given her hatred of doctors and her dependence on alcohol. She wore an old threadbare Arsenal replica shirt from the early-1990s' George Graham era; her wasted arms were heavily tattooed. (I could read one, which proclaimed: 'Only God can judge me'.) 'You're just going to fuck me out the door without sorting me out,' she spat. You're probably right, I thought. She discharged herself later that day 'against medical advice'.

An Englishman with alcoholic cirrhosis had been transferred the day before from the small county hospital in west Cork; he had a huge mane of grey hair and a full, Old Testament prophet beard. (I have often been struck by the sheer hairiness of men with liver cirrhosis: you hardly ever see a bald one.) West Cork was full of retired English people, a migration that had always puzzled me. I suspect they arrived as tourists on a sunny summer's day, became intoxicated with the scenery and the charm of the locals, and as soon as they were back home in Doncaster or Croydon, they were looking at Irish properties online. Before they knew it, they were in Kealkill, staring out at the rain on a wet November Wednesday, wondering what had possessed them. It's no wonder they took to drink.

Alan was on a trolley in the emergency department. He was now thirty-five; I had known him since he was a teenager. His case notes were in five telephone-directory-sized volumes; he had been attending the ministry since both he and the institution were in their infancy. He had spent at least half his life here and over the years had developed a weary cynicism in his dealings with doctors. Fixing me with his watery eyes, Alan asked: 'What's causing this pain?' He might as well have asked me to explain quantum mechanics.

To the surgical ward, to see another cirrhotic woman, Colette. Only thirty, she was so jaundiced her skin colour had progressed from yellow to *green*. With a sublime disregard for her plight, she announced that she would go home. I told her that if she did so she would die, but I wouldn't stop her from leaving. My lack of opposition – indeed indifference – to this threat was paradoxically effective, for she made no further mention of it. The nurses asked me whether they should call security if she tried to bolt; I told them she had the capacity to make her own decisions, and that no obstacles should be placed in her path. The senior nurse didn't disguise her disapproval of this: 'What if she dies?' She would die anyway, I thought, here or at home, now or later. But that wasn't what worried her; she had visions of a newspaper headline: 'Woman fatally injured by lorry minutes after absconding from hospital'.

Delusions of competence

Every Monday morning, Terence, head of the health and well-being service for the southern region, sent an email to 'all users' with his 'weekly wellbeing messages'. There were always three: one on 'spirituality', a second on exercise and a third on diet. Did Terence deliberately choose Monday morning to send these messages – thinking it the time when we coalface health workers would be in most need of his encouragement? Here are this week's suggestions:

- Accept your flaws, they make you *you*
- Dance like no one is watching
- Eat a pear a day

Terence started sending these messages early in 2019. His many 'spiritual' exhortations included: be thankful for what you have; lending an ear is lending a hand; rest to recharge your batteries; do something kind for someone today; ask your colleagues how you can help them; tell someone you are proud of them; appreciate the world; list five things you are happy about; three hugs a day; forgive and forget; stop comparing yourself to others; give somebody a compliment; give yourself credit for your achievements; do more of what you love; be open to new ideas; surround yourself with positive people; appreciate the beauty of nature; learn from your mistakes; spend time with those who you love; recognise your strengths; be proud of who you are; be kind to yourself; keep a positive attitude; don't take tomorrow to bed with you; laugh more; make a new friend; be your own best friend; do not fear change; live in the moment.

I almost looked forward to these banalities; they eased me into the week. I had a vision of Terence at his desk in the Skibbereen office of Cork-Kerry Community Healthcare, his desk groaning with books by Deepak Chopra, Paulo Coelho and the Dalai Lama, wondering what messages to send every week. My colleague David, however, viewed Terence's dietary tips ('practise mindful eating') as dangerous nonsense. When Terence advised 'all users' to 'be sure to drink 2 litres of water per day', David was infuriated enough to email me:

> 'Be sure to drink 2 litres of water per day.' Unless, of course, you (1) Don't trust your own highly sensitive thirst regulation; (2) Have chronic heart failure; (3) Have psychogenic polydipsia; (4) Think that it is strongly evidence-based; (5) Drink too much of it; (6) Think that you will lose weight by it; and (7) Don't mind the odd bug.

'These messages are such hogwash,' he wrote, 'and not as harmless as they seem.' I replied to David that while I agreed with him, he should *really* write to Terence with these concerns.

A woman was 'handed back' to me over the weekend: she had been admitted under another physician, but because she had been under our service (with a completely unrelated problem) within the previous six months, we were obliged – by the ancient rules governing medical 'take' – to accept her back under *our* care. She was suffering such severe alcohol withdrawal that she required not only large doses of sedatives but also the continuous presence of a 'special' – in this instance, a burly African care assistant – to prevent her from hurting herself or any of the staff, and to stop her from defenestrating. A psychiatrist suggested a stint in a rehabilitation unit. She told him that she didn't have any confidence in this unit.

'Why is that?' he asked.

'Because I worked there as a counsellor.' Did she lack confidence in this unit because she knew from her experience there that it wasn't very good, or because they were foolish enough to hire someone as troubled as her?

When I saw her the next day, she seemed greatly improved. She talked warmly of her home village and her GP. This conversation went on for some time before my registrar whispered to me: 'She's not our patient.' This new woman now occupied the same single room where my alcoholic addiction counsellor had been 'specialled'; *she* had been transferred overnight to another ward. I hadn't caught a very good view of her the day before, curled up in a ball, hidden beneath the bedclothes while she weathered the horrors of *delirium tremens*.

*

Alan, the full-time patient who was on a trolley in the emergency department when I last saw him, was now languishing on a surgical ward. An on-call junior doctor had, for some unfathomable reason – probably at the prompting of a dietician – requested blood phosphate levels on Alan. His phosphate levels were low, which led to several intravenous phosphate infusions, with little effect on his pain or his mood. Someone else had ordered an MRI scan of his liver, but this could not be done because Alan had metal somewhere in his ravaged body.* Now he wanted to know why he was so deficient in phosphate and why couldn't he have the MRI? After a long conversation with him, I took the registrar and senior house officer aside.

'Alan is a *super-tanker*,' I explained. 'Super-tankers can have only one *captain*, one doctor who makes any significant decisions. Alan's captain is not "on" for the wards right now, so we should do as little as possible. Preferably nothing.'

⌇

I greeted the *hospitaleras*† on the main corridor: that small group of older women who, despite having no official appointment or institutional recognition, spent most of their days in the

---

* MRI scanners use strong magnets, which can cause migration and heating of metal implants.

† I borrowed this from the Spanish word for the volunteers who assist pilgrims on the Camino to Santiago de Compostela. The original medieval *hospitaleros* were pilgrims who never went home.

ministry. They ate in the canteen and attended daily mass in the chapel. I nodded to each in turn; I knew them all.

When the ministry opened, you could smoke almost anywhere: in the canteen, in the ward day rooms, in the medical students' locker room, in the junior doctors' lounge, in the surgeons' coffee room, in theatre. 'We must stop for a smoke,' one registrar who worked at the ministry in the 1980s would *order* her willing consultant, mid-ward round. This saturnine, elegant man would then join her for a cigarette in the ward sister's office. Even the shop on the main corridor sold cigarettes. Now the smokers were banished, and you could no more buy tobacco in the ministry than you could a bottle of whiskey. Staff who were smokers either went out to the main road, to a corner adjoining a suburban street, or to their cars, which, strictly speaking, was not allowed, since the entire campus was now non-smoking. There were still a few smoking doctors; one didn't bother to skulk: he puffed insouciantly in the ambulance bay by the emergency department.

Because our department (offices, secretaries and outpatient clinic) was housed in a building near the periphery of the campus, I walked through the main entrance several times every day on my way to the wards or the endoscopy unit. The drug reps, with their tight suits and shiny brown shoes, congregated just inside the door, while outside were the smokers. They gathered in a comradely huddle, often sheltering from wind and rain, in their pyjamas and dressing gowns. Some carried urinary catheter bags; others grasped their drip stands, like the figures from Géricault's *Raft of the Medusa* clinging to the mast of the raft.* Immediately above the ministry entrance, a public address system played an announcement on a continuous loop. The voice (with an English accent – still the sound of authority in Ireland) admonished them for exposing the patients in the breast and cardiac units to their second-hand smoke.

Middle-class families walked or cycled through the ministry grounds on their way to the local schools. Some of the parents were 'presentational' – their conversations with their children meant for a wider audience: 'Cian, Sadhbh: *that's* a blackbird; the other one is a jackdaw!' A few cycled behind their children, like the *domestiques* in the Tour de France.

* Géricault used to visit the Beaujon Hospital in Paris to sketch dying patients as models for these figures; 'nothing repulsed him,' wrote the art historian Georges-Antoine Borias. He painted several lunatics, most notably *Man with Delusions of Military Rank*. I fantasised about commissioning a portrait of a colleague, entitled *Doctor with Delusions of Competence*.

Felix

The building that housed the gastroenterology outpatient clinic was near the back entrance of the ministry. Although this outpatient clinic had been specially established for that group of women who had been infected with the hepatitis C virus after receiving the anti-D vaccine,* the ministry agreed that all the other liver and gastroenterology outpatient clinics could also be held there. The main hospital outpatients was shared by many different departments, but this clinic was *ours*: we had our own nurses and receptionists; the waiting area and four consultation rooms were bright and spacious;

* Anti-D vaccine is routinely given to pregnant women who are negative for the rhesus blood type to prevent rhesus disease, where the mother makes antibodies against the baby's red blood cells. In 1994, it was discovered that two batches of anti-D vaccine given to pregnant women in Ireland during the late 1970s and early 1990s, respectively, were contaminated with the hepatitis C virus, which can cause chronic liver disease. Over 1,200 women were found to be infected. This was probably the greatest of the many scandals in Irish health care since the foundation of the state. Five special clinics (three in Dublin, one each in Cork and Galway) were established to care for these 'state-infected' women.

the two secretaries and four consultants had their offices there also.

Felix, the first patient that day at the clinic, had chronic abdominal pain. His name only drew ironic attention to his gloomy disposition; Felix lived in a hell of his designing. I had investigated this pain extensively, finding no cause. 'Yer doin' nathin' for me,' he said in his drawling monotone. I reassured him that all the tests were clear, and that this was *good*. Felix was not consoled: 'Yer hidin' somethin' from me. I know ye are. There's somethin' awful wrong with me.'

An urgent email from a middle-ranking manager, the 'lead for unscheduled care':

The hospital is in the highest level of escalation this morning with 27 patients in the ED [emergency department], 12 patients in the AMAU [acute medical assessment unit] and 7 patients across the main wards who have not been allocated a bed. This is the case due to low number of discharges over the weekend. Including the 21 elective admissions this morning who also need beds, there is a requirement for 66 beds as we start the day.

In order to de-escalate the hospital the Flow Team need to have early visibility of potential discharges.

> There were 45 potential discharges highlighted at 9 am
> and this does not meet the current demand.

The management narrative – a cynically clever one – was that the 'trolley' crisis* was due to 'low number of discharges over the weekend', *not* an inadequate number of beds. If only the consultants could be bothered to come in at weekends and *discharge* patients, we would not be faced with this problem on Monday: the doctors had failed to *maximise patient flow*.

⌒

Tim, the radiologist who chaired our weekly X-ray conference, was away; nobody could deputise for him, because the radiology department was 'swamped'. This meeting was important. Tim reviewed X-rays and scans of patients we had concerns about; not infrequently, he overturned the diagnosis of his radiology colleagues. Many – if not most – of the weekly conferences like this (particularly those held over lunchtime) were 'sponsored' by the pharmaceutical industry, who supplied food and drinks. I had long since declined this largesse; none of my colleagues shared my unease. A drug rep stood forlorn by the sandwiches and tins of Diet Cola he had provided for this meeting, which would now not proceed.

---

* This 'crisis' had continued for many years, even decades. Because the ministry (and most other hospitals like it in Ireland) did not have enough beds to accommodate the ever-growing demands for inpatient care, patients presenting to the emergency department who were deemed to require admission to hospital often spent many hours – sometimes *days* – on trolleys in that department, while they awaited a bed.

One of my colleagues instructed the juniors to eat the sponsored lunch; it was, he said, 'the least we could do'.

⌒

On call today, general medical 'take'. I took a call from a locum consultant at a small private hospital sixty miles away. He spoke for some time about an elderly male patient; all I could ascertain from this monologue was that he wanted to transfer him as quickly as possible.

'What do you think is wrong with him?' I asked.

'I don't know, but he needs multidisciplinary care.' I could sense his desperation. 'Multidisciplinary care' was clearly something not provided by this private hospital. I explained to this doctor that I would do my best to find a bed for his patient at the ministry, but given the fact that over twenty patients were being accommodated on trolleys in the emergency department, it was unlikely that I would be able to get the patient in that evening. I asked him to email me the patient's details; I never heard from him again.

I wasn't disturbed overnight, a great relief, since being woken by a call from the ministry had become increasingly onerous. I found it nearly impossible to make rational decisions after being shocked out of a deep slumber, and often struggled to get back to sleep. As usual after a night on call, I got up at 5.30, breakfasted in my office at 6.30, and started at 7.00 in the emergency department, where most of my patients would be accommodated in cubicles or on trolleys. I struggled, as always, to find somewhere wide enough and flat enough to write in the notes, and a clean, empty sink in which to wash my hands between patients.

An elderly woman lying on a trolley with a fractured pelvis and collarbone (sustained after a fall), cellulitis and septicaemia looked ghastly. Her husband and daughter hovered anxiously, while a nurse told me, in a loud whisper, 'Her blood pressure is dropping!' Having delivered this message, she walked off.

A man with heart failure. He was only sixty-two, but this was his third admission in six months. He attended several services (respiratory, cardiology, diabetes). Who would have the difficult conversation with him? Who will tell him that he won't survive another year?

A floater

When I drove in, there were pickets at the hospital gates; the non-clinical support staff were on strike. I talked to a porter on the picket line. The money needed to settle their grievance was about 10 per cent of the sum spent on resolving a recent dispute with the consultants.

⌒

I noticed a 'floater' in my left eye: a jagged crack in my peripheral vision. I phoned my ophthalmologist friend Sam, who saw me immediately in his private rooms. The vitreous (jelly) had peeled off the retina, 'like an orange', according to Sam. There was nothing to be done, he said, apart from regular checks to make sure the retina hadn't detached, which would be much more serious.

⌒

The first patient at the clinic was a woman who had had swallowing difficulty (dysphagia) for years. Now in her late sixties, her file was large. I found a note I had written when I was a senior house officer in 1984, confirming that she was 'medically fit for discharge' after taking an overdose. I was tempted to mention that we'd met before, but decided it might be best not to. People rarely like to be reminded of such incidents from their distant past.

The next man also had dysphagia. His GP wrote that he was 'very concerned' that he might have oesophageal cancer and requested an urgent appointment. The patient had visited this GP to get a routine prescription renewed and mentioned that he sometimes noticed he had difficulty swallowing. 'I tried to tell him that it was because my dentures had loosened, but he wouldn't listen.' This doctor knew that the word 'dysphagia' in the referral letter would trigger an urgent appointment, regardless of whether the patient's dysphagia was caused by oesophageal cancer or ill-fitting dentures.

The first patient I saw on my ward round that afternoon was a ninety-four-year-old nun who had been admitted with a stomach bleed. Sister Walburga had dementia and was sent in from her nursing home. A few years before, when she was still *compos mentis*, she had completed an advance care directive,* stating that she wanted *everything*: cardio-pulmonary resuscitation, ventilation in the intensive care unit, PEG tube-feeding,† dialysis. Some patients thought these directives were like a menu ('yes, I'll have the PEG tube, the chemotherapy and the ventilation, but I'll pass on the dialysis'), but all they can legally do is clarify for doctors what you *don't* want. Another doctor had placed a DNACPR (do not attempt cardio-pulmonary resuscitation) notice in her chart a year before; I saw no reason to remove it. But I wondered why a *religious* person was so desperate to cling on to life at ninety, so reluctant to meet her maker. Was Sister Walburga having a late-life crisis of faith? Did she no longer believe in the life eternal and the communion of saints?

The woman with the fractured pelvis and septicaemia whom I had seen the day before in the emergency department was much better. I asked about the accident.

'A young fella ran into me in the street and knocked me over.'

'Did he stop?'

'Indeed then he did not.'

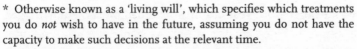

* Otherwise known as a 'living will', which specifies which treatments you do *not* wish to have in the future, assuming you do not have the capacity to make such decisions at the relevant time.

† PEG (percutaneous endoscopic gastrostomy): a feeding tube placed endoscopically directly into the stomach through the abdominal wall.

The bed managers obsessed about the 'whiteboards', magnetic noticeboards mounted on every ward, which were supposed to alert all 'stakeholders' to which patients were ready for discharge, who was awaiting a scan, and so on. We doctors were obliged to estimate the 'planned discharge date' of our patients; without this information, the bed managers told us, they couldn't manage patient *flow*. The bed office sent this choleric email to all the consultants:

> We hope you can understand that it is IMPOSSIBLE to plan where admitted patients in the Emergency Depart–ment will go when we have <u>no visibility for discharges.</u> <u>Tracking daily flow is the first point in being able to plan</u> <u>flow and escalate issues.</u> We can only do our job if we have the support of staff on the wards to guide us about each patient's journey. We really need your help.

I struggled with the concept of the 'planned discharge date'; I could not predict with any accuracy the date of my patients' departure as if they were hotel guests. How long would Sister Walburga need? I couldn't say.

I attended a compulsory training session on the white-board; the clinical director* turned up to make sure all the consultants were there. Two managers explained the codes for the coloured magnetic discs. There were five colour codes relating to discharge and four for tests and interventions. 'Whiteboards,' said the smiling quality improvement manager,

---

* Clinical directors are hospital consultants who have a managerial role. They are meant to act as a conduit between senior hospital management and the doctors.

'are not a substitute for staff speaking to each other', but that was precisely what they were. Relatives looked at the boards too; one enterprising family deduced that one of the coloured discs next to their mother's name was the code for 'palliative care'. They didn't know until then that she was dying.

'Jesus, has anyone got a fag?'

I went to the eye clinic for a check-up. I had a long wait. So this is what it's like to be a patient. Waiting. Not Knowing. Unlike other clinics in the hospital, we all sat, not in a waiting room, but on benches outside the consulting rooms. Two men – one very old, one late middle-aged – sat together near me; it was difficult to tell which was the 'carer'. It reminded me of a patient, a man in his late nineties with a tight oesophageal stricture (narrowing of the gullet). He was reluctant to come in to have this stricture dilated (stretched), he told me, because there was no one else to look after his seventy-year-old son.

Waiting with me was a retired surgeon; I was once his intern. I recalled the weekly teaching conference in the early 1980s, when the surgeons and their teams gathered in the windowless tutorial room near the ward. At one such meeting, a nurse brought in a patient, a shaven-headed man in his forties, wearing pyjamas. Two prongs were sticking out of his head: these were ventricular drains to relieve hydrocephalus (fluid on the brain). 'He looks like a Martian,' one of the surgeons joked, loud enough for the man to hear; his steroid-bloated face bore an expression of infinite sadness and defiant dignity.

The surgeon had been the ministry's chairman of medical staff in the late 1980s. His greatest achievement in this role, to his mind, was blocking the erection of a statue of Padre Pio* on the front lawn of the hospital. He quite correctly argued that because the ministry was *not* a Catholic-run institution, such a memorial would be inappropriate.

The Capuchin friar had a great following in Ireland at that time: many cars displayed a windscreen sticker with his image, believed to protect the driver from accidents. Holy man he may have been, but I always thought Padre Pio had a menacing, malicious look about him – more Irish peasant than Italian mystic. It's the dark eyes and caterpillar eyebrows, I think.

When the ministry opened in 1978, it may have been under municipal control – and therefore officially secular – but its ethos was nevertheless strongly Catholic. Nuns occupied nearly all the senior nursing posts, such as matron and head of the school of nursing. The spacious Catholic chapel was dedicated to 'Christ our Saviour', vastly grander than the tiny, humble Anglican chapel of 'Christ the Healer' around the corner. The Vienna Boys' Choir sang in the chapel of Christ

---

* Padre Pio (1887–1968) was a celebrated Italian priest and stigmatist, alleged bearer of the bleeding wounds of Christ. Pio is reputed to have restored the sight of a blind Sicilian girl, Gemma di Giorgi, in 1947. In 1956 he established a hospital (*Casa Sollievo della Sofferenza*) in San Giovanni Rotondo, in Foggia, southern Italy. He was canonised in 2002.

our Saviour in November 1979; a Mr Kenneth Jones worked through the night to install the piped organ for their concert.

Now, nobody much cared about Padre Pio. In one generation, the Irish had gone from pious lickspittles to aggressive secularists. I almost missed the nuns. Forty years on, an ever-dwindling, ever-ageing congregation of people who lived nearby turned up for Sunday mass in the chapel of Christ our Saviour, more an act of habit than one of worship. Muslim worshippers now outnumbered the Christians; the ministry employed so many Pakistani doctors that a temporary Islamic prayer room – fashioned from an old steel freight container – was installed on the ministry grounds. The only available space was near the mortuary.

In the 1980s, the Catholic chaplain on duty was part of the cardiac arrest team. I was on call one evening when the arrest call went out from the haematology ward. This ward also housed the burns unit, and always reeked of burnt flesh. A young leukaemia patient had had a cardiac arrest; after thirty minutes of futile and bloody work, the medical registrar called 'enough'. In those days, we didn't engage in difficult conversations about resuscitation and 'ceiling of care';* this young

* This term means a predetermined highest level of intervention deemed appropriate by doctors, in line (if possible) with the wishes of the patient and family. The term is often used when making decisions about cardio-pulmonary resuscitation (CPR) and admission to intensive care for ventilation. The very use of the term 'ceiling of care' by doctors usually means that they believe such interventions to be futile.

man's leukaemia was well beyond any hope of cure by the time his heart stopped beating. We stood there, silent and ashamed, the lifeless bruised body on the bed, the floor covered with discarded needles and syringes. The door burst open: the chaplain, a stocky country boy of thirty, came in, panting, red-faced, smelling of alcohol. He anointed the corpse and said some short prayers. When he had completed his sacerdotal duties, he sighed: 'Jesus, has anyone got a fag?'

Sam, my eye doctor, was weary when he finally got to me. The vitreous detachment was unchanged, the retina was intact. He would, however, need to see me every week until the end of the month. Was this standard practice, I wondered, or was he being excessively cautious, wary about treating a colleague? He explained everything to me in some detail. I told him: 'Sam, I trust you. Do what you think is right.' I was tempted to add: 'Just be *paternalistic*.'

The new paradigm of the doctor-patient relationship was 'shared decision-making': the physician's role was to summarise all the options, risks and benefits, and to support the patient in whatever decision he or she made. This new model was based on a flawed assumption, namely, that people think and behave in the same way when they are sick as they do when in the full of their health. Two years before, when I was admitted to the coronary care unit, I was as weak and dependent as a baby; what surprised me was that I did not rebel against this vulnerability. I simply wanted the doctors and nurses to look after me. The cardiologist who attended me was naturally anxious to discuss the technical aspects of my investigations and treatment, more than he would have done with a 'lay' person. To my surprise, I had no curiosity about these matters; I told him to do whatever he thought was best. It wasn't that I was indifferent – I was anxious to recover – but I didn't want information, choices, agency, control; I simply wanted to feel safe, comforted.

Even the most self-reliant individuals feel like this when they become sick. When Evelyn Waugh went mad in 1954,* he was convinced that he was 'possessed', and begged his friend, the Jesuit priest Father Philip Caraman, to exorcise him. Caraman instead wisely summoned the psychiatrist Eric Strauss.† Waugh, recalled Caraman, 'was just like a child in his hands. He answered every question Dr Strauss asked him as though he was a schoolboy. He had great confidence in him.' Strauss ordered Waugh to stop taking the sedative drugs chloral and bromide (which he had been using for his chronic insomnia), gave him instead paraldehyde, and his hallucinations ceased.

* Suffering from fatigue and chronic ill health, Waugh embarked on a sea voyage to Ceylon in January 1954, hoping that this break would restore his vitality. During this journey, he experienced a psychotic break-down, with disturbing auditory hallucinations. This episode inspired his novel *The Ordeal of Gilbert Pinfold*.

† E.B. Strauss (1894–1961) was a psychiatrist at St Bartholomew's Hospital, London. His obituary in the *British Medical Journal* described him thus: 'E. B. Strauss had a fine presence and a personality compounded of grace, gentleness, dignity, courtesy, wisdom and learning. He had considerable charm of personality, a rich and soothing voice, and a quiet playful sense of humour. He looked distinguished, especially when sporting his familiar monocle.' Unusual for a psychoanalyst at that time, Strauss was a devout Catholic. Little wonder Waugh placed himself so willingly in his care.

Icians and Ologists

I began my round in the emergency department. My first patient was a woman on a trolley. Her belly was drum-tight with fluid retention caused by liver disease; the trolley barely contained her bulk. She was sobbing loudly, her huge body shuddering.

On my home ward, a patient of mine with chronic liver disease had a nasogastric feeding tube inserted; I hadn't ordered this. The registrar and senior house officer sheepishly told me that a dietician had told them to do it, because she had calculated that he was 'not meeting his caloric requirements'. I found no pressing reason for this tube-feeding and told them to remove it. This instruction was met with much eyebrow-raising.

A woman in the intensive care unit had shot off half of her face in a botched suicide attempt. The doctors there wanted us to insert a PEG feeding tube; luckily, she didn't need this. The ministry was now as assiduous in keeping her alive as she had been maladroit in her attempt to kill herself.

E. B. Strauss was mystified that suicide was relatively uncommon: 'Why is it then, that so few of us, numerically speaking, commit suicide, in spite of the fact that so many of us suffer severe reverses of fortune in the course of our lives and are called upon at various times to put up with almost intolerable pain?'

When we broke for tea at the canteen midway through the round, my registrar told me about the 'live' endoscopy demonstration he had attended in Amsterdam. He gave me a breathless account of the complex and super-specialised procedures he had witnessed, such as the endoscopic removal of huge colonic polyps and superficial gastric cancers. I had once, before I came back to the ministry, seen myself as the kind of doctor who carried out such technical feats.

There are two kinds of doctor: icians and ologists, such as geriatr-*icians* and ophthalm-*ologists*. Ologists belong to the Asclepian* tradition, which focuses on the specific causes of disease, while icians – supposedly – adhere to the Hygieian† tradition, which regards health as being in harmony with oneself and one's environment. The real difference, if I am to be truthful, is that icians are *low status* and ologists are *high status*.

* Asclepius was the Greek god of medicine.
† Hygieia was the Greek goddess of good health.

I trained to be an ologist, but I was now (mainly) an ician. This was not intentional, not a conversion. I came back to the ministry in 2001, full of notions about interventional endoscopy, thinking myself an elite super-technician. After the first week, I knew that dream was over. I inherited a neglected, demoralised service, which for several years had trundled along, just surviving. On the first ward round, I saw a woman who had been in for a long time.

'How long has she been in?' I asked the registrar.

After much scrutiny of the notes, he replied: 'Thirteen months.'

'Why is she still here?'

'I don't know.'

I became an ician, a generalist and a palliator, because that was what the job required. My work was much nearer to psychiatry or general practice than it was to, say, ophthalmology. I mourned the super-technician, the ologist. I was now an ician, combining elements of priest, social worker and counsellor. Icians bumble along, bring the patient back to the clinic every three months, fill in death certificates and – if brave enough – have difficult conversations with patients and relatives. Icians are water carriers, bearers of responsibility, the name on the sticker.* Bullied by managers and clinical directors, they rarely cure anyone. Ologists, however,

* Whenever a patient was admitted to the ministry, stickers were printed with details of the person's name, address, date of birth, hospital number and responsible consultant. These stickers were attached to forms for X-rays and blood tests, saving time on handwriting and reducing – supposedly – clerical errors. 'The name on the sticker' became my personal shorthand for clinical responsibility; I would remind the junior doctors that apart from the patient's, there was only one name on the sticker: *mine.*

are usually faced with a single problem to *fix*. They regard the word 'holistic' with scorn; can you imagine a discipline called the *orthopaedic humanities?*

Some icians have managed to partly reconfigure themselves as ologists. Several geriatricians, for example, now called themselves 'stroke physicians'. When thrombectomy* came along as a treatment for acute stroke, and was shown to work, they suddenly had at their disposal a highly effective, technically challenging intervention, which had a narrow window of opportunity (four hours from the onset of symptoms). Even though the tricky stuff (the *actual* removal of the blood clot from the brain) was done by neuroradiologists, the 'stroke physicians' started to swagger like heart surgeons, telling the rest of us that with this treatment, 'every second counts'.

I still did a little ologist work; very occasionally, I was a patient's ician *and* ologist. A man who came under my care with a fractured pelvis was astonished when, a week after he came in, I removed – endoscopically – the bile duct stones that gave him septicaemia. It's as if your social worker called round to fix your central heating or to do the conveyancing on the sale of your house.

⌣⟩

* The radiologically guided removal of a fresh blood clot from the brain in stroke patients. The neuroradiologist punctures the femoral artery in the groin and passes a tube into the arteries in the brain. The blood clot causing the stroke is caught by a stent-like device, and then retrieved, with restoration of the blood supply and reversal of the paralysis. This procedure is available only in large centres.

I gave €50 to my intern as my contribution to the annual interns' party. I never went, but some of the consultants did, hoping that by the time the party moved from the pub to the rugby club, there would be a temporary Saturnalian suspension of hierarchical professional boundaries. This annual event used to be held in the hospital but was banned sometime in the 1990s after one riotous event, involving several now highly respectable doctors and the police. Middle-aged male doctors love to be the subject of such rumours and urban myths; they stiffen with pride when suspected of being a salty old dog. Saltiest by far of these old dogs were the 'alickadoos' who attached themselves as non-playing members of the university rugby club. They went on tour with 'the boys', tidying up after them, paying off the hotels.

An email announced the retirement of a manager. She entered the ministry as a student nurse, and apart from six weeks in Dublin at a residential course on 'leadership', she spent the next forty years there. She was cunning and resilient, and remembered every slight, real or imagined. She was leaving, she said, to 'pursue new challenges in the private sector'.

'You'll do'

The first patient at that morning's clinic was a man of seventy-eight with a full head of dyed red hair, framing a wizened, aged face. He told me he hadn't eaten *anything* in six weeks. He wasn't pleased when I told him that he hadn't lost any weight since his last visit.

A woman with chronic diarrhoea who had attended me for years arrived with a printout documenting her bowel movements over the six months since her last appointment, along with a typed list of her 'Main Symptoms':

Recurrent pain in the lower abdomen region. The pain varies from a dull ache to a strong spasm type. Persistent diarrhoea often with little or no warning. Multiple bowel openings during the day and night. Feeling of nausea with bouts of sickness. Sudden onset of feeling very tired and listless. Sudden change in complexion to a yellow or very pale colour. Aches in the ankles and the right shoulder. Also in the fingers. Food passes through the system in a matter of an hour or so usually mostly undigested. Peas appear to be the worst food that produces this event although other greens have no notable effect. I have noticed that there is a tendency to feel the need for a bowel evacuation during or soon after eating. Recurrent inflammation of the eyes. The prescribed eye drops have little or no effect. During the last six months I have experienced an increase in difficulty to sleep at night. I awaken gasping for breath as though my chest is being pressed down. Due to the nature of the bowel evacuations I have been unable to leave my house for several years unless I prepare by fasting for a couple of days and then taking Imodium. This does not remove the problem completely and always has a price to pay later. I have not been out from my home apart from the test in hospital this year.

I read this document carefully, pausing occasionally to clarify a detail. I had long since given up trying to nudge her in a 'psychological' direction. Her diarrhoea was caused by irritable bowel syndrome (IBS),* the commonest diagnosis made at my clinic. The most neurotic of these patients had constellations of other, non-gut symptoms, so they often attended several clinics, as indeed did this woman. Patients with such multiple 'medically unexplained symptoms' were usually given the label of 'somatisation disorder', which was deemed to be

* Symptoms of IBS include cramping, bloating, flatulence, and diarrhoea or constipation, or both. Because it is a 'syndrome' (as opposed to a 'disease'), investigations such as colonoscopy and CT scans are normal.

less offensive and judgemental than 'psychosomatic'. My role was to listen, to contain, to gently disabuse her of her most delusional and outlandish beliefs.

Medical manpower phoned in the middle of clinic. I was on call for general medicine that night, and one of the house officers rostered to be on duty phoned in sick; none of her colleagues would cover. Manpower were calling, they explained, 'just to let you know'. I instantly regretted giving €50 to the interns' party.

I sensed things were bad when I came in at 7.00 the next morning. A distracted senior house officer handed me a list of twenty new patients. An alcoholic man who came in with seizures was comatose and Cheyne-Stoking.* Three nurses suddenly appeared and rushed the man into the resus room,† where they commenced CPR. I stood there, watching them at work, feeling foolish and quite useless.

---

* Cheyne-Stokes respiration is a pattern of breathing typically seen in the dying. The breathing becomes progressively faster and deeper, then briefly stops, only for the cycle to start again. John Cheyne (1777–1836) was a Scot who worked in Dublin from 1811 to 1831; William Stokes (1804–78) was Irish. The surgeon and poet Oliver St John Gogarty wrote this doggerel: *They were a fearless nation / whose only hesitation / was Cheyne-Stokes respiration.*

† The resus (resuscitation) room of the emergency department is where the sickest patients were accommodated.

*

Over tea, my registrar told me – almost as an afterthought – that an elderly female patient of mine, who was awaiting placement in a nursing home, had died over the weekend. She had developed an acute bowel obstruction; while the surgeons dithered about operating, she aspirated into her lungs and died choking on her own vomit. The attrition rate of those 'awaiting long-term care' was alarmingly high.

'What about the family?' I asked nervously.

'Oh, there's no near relatives,' he said. I was relieved. Even though I had no involvement in the events of the weekend, I might still – as the patient's consultant, the *name* on the hospital sticker – have to answer any awkward questions from relatives about the circumstances of her death.

After tea, we saw a man in the intensive care unit who had taken an overdose of sleeping tablets and blood pressure pills. When he was brought into the emergency department, he was so comatose that he was taken to the unit and ventilated overnight. He had woken up. Although intent on killing himself only the day before, he was now anxious to be seen by a cardiologist: 'I've been getting this vague chest discomfort and I'm very worried it could be angina.'

We went back to the emergency department to see a woman admitted under cardiology the night before by a junior doctor who thought the patient's breathlessness was caused by heart failure. They now refused to take her, saying she did *not* have

45

heart failure, so she had to go to general medicine, which was me. She was lying on a trolley in the back corridor of the emergency department, talking on her phone, telling her interlocutor: 'I'm waiting for the cardiologist.' I introduced myself and explained that the cardiologists didn't want her, and that she would have to come under my care. 'You'll do,' she said sweetly.

The liver queen

I did two endoscopy lists every week; a decade before, I often did *four*. A list lasted about four hours, during which I carried out a mix of gastroscopies and colonoscopies. A gastroscopy usually took about five minutes, which led to frequent requests for 'a *quick* scope'. I sedated the patients with a mixture of midazolam (a Valium-like drug) and fentanyl (an opiate now often mentioned in the context of the epidemic in the US). Gastroscopies are mainly done to investigate indigestion ('dyspepsia'), and are, indeed, usually 'quick'. Once the patient was adequately sedated (the determination of which is an inexact science), I gently passed the black flexible endoscope (width of a little finger) through the mouth, over the tongue, through the pharynx (throat) into the oesophagus (gullet). When performed in patients with bleeding from the stomach or oesophagus, however, gastroscopy can be time-consuming and technically demanding, with therapeutic interventions such as injection of stomach ulcers and the placement of rubber bands ('banding') around varicose veins in the oesophagus.

A colonoscopy takes much longer to perform than a gastroscopy – usually twenty to thirty minutes. It is also a much greater undertaking for the patients, because they must consume large quantities of laxative fluid to cleanse the bowel. The main challenge for the doctor performing the procedure is the removal of polyps. These are benign, berry-like growths in the bowel, which are usually removed, because some of them – over many years – may become cancerous. Removal of these polyps can sometimes cause complications of bleeding and bowel perforation. As time went on, I had become increasingly fearful of such 'adverse events', having experienced most of them over the years. I consoled myself with the endoscopists' mantra: that a doctor who has never caused these complications is a doctor who hasn't done enough procedures.

The endoscopy procedure with the greatest risk is ERCP (endoscopic retrograde cholangio-pancreatography), used to remove gallstones from the bile duct, and to insert stents through cancerous blockages. ERCP-related complications (pancreatitis, bleeding, infection) are sometimes life-threatening, and, very rarely, fatal. I was proud that I had brought this procedure to the ministry, but when, years later, a newly appointed colleague expressed a desire to take over, I handed over my list to him without regret. I had had enough.

That afternoon, I carried out a colonoscopy on a man who, when he came to see me at the clinic some weeks before, was very anxious to let me know about his social connections with senior doctors in the hospital. He managed to convey this before any discussion of his symptoms. Oh yes, he played golf with X, he went sailing with Y. The Irish assume that unless you insinuate yourself with a professional, unless you obligate them with some tenuous social connection, they won't do a 'proper' job. An Englishman, I thought, would never do this.

⌒

Anticipating another long wait at the eye clinic, I brought a book with me, a biography of Professor Dame Sheila Sherlock. Sherlock (1918–2001) was a pioneer in liver disease, and the first woman in Britain (indeed, in *Europe*) to become a full professor of medicine when she was appointed to the chair at the Royal Free Hospital in London in 1959. The worse she treated them, the more her 'boys' – her many registrars and research fellows – adored her. They couldn't get enough of her: the bullying, the sarcasm, the single-mindedness. Her obituary in the *British Medical Journal* reported that 'she reduced male junior doctors to tears'. This biography, written by one these acolytes – one Om P. Sharma – is obsequiously entitled *Prof: The Life of Sheila Sherlock 'The liver queen'*. Awful stuff – 'Under a somewhat tart manner, Sheila had a sensitive heart' – but no period of history, as they say, is more interesting than the recent past.

Sherlock was a brilliant woman who carried out ground-breaking research in liver disease at the Hammersmith Hospital in the 1940s and '50s. She subjected hundreds of patients – who did not know they were being used as guinea pigs – to potentially dangerous procedures such as liver biopsy, solely for research purposes. When another doctor raised concerns about her activities, she told him: 'This is what happens, this is what I do. Don't be such a silly old fogey.' I do not suppose she ever entertained a moment of self-doubt. A photograph of the academic medical staff at the Hammersmith taken in the 1940s shows a group of eighteen sitting around a dinner table. At the head of the table is the chief of medicine, Sir John McMichael; on his right sits Sherlock, head thrown back, imperiously gazing at the camera, the only woman: 'Sheila in the Den of Lions'. Like Margaret Thatcher, she was *not* a feminist. How anaemic and biddable our contemporary academic 'leaders' seem in comparison.

'Sheila Sherlock never bore a grudge,' Sharma writes. A useful attribute, I thought, not bearing grudges. I have only accrued enemies; once I made an enemy, they stayed an enemy: they never returned to the ranks of non-enemies, ex-enemies, or – God forbid – friends. They only deepened, like Larkin's coastal shelf. I have nursed grudges like others have cellared fine old wines.

'Is there anything to be said for another mass?'

Although I wasn't on call, I came in over the weekend to see a sick patient. I noticed that the woman in the next bed was looking at me intently. This often happens in medicine; over the years, you see thousands of people and it can be difficult to recognise them later, out of context. I knew I had seen her before, but I couldn't remember when or for what. When she said: 'I'm Patricia's mother', I knew immediately.

Patricia had died of alcoholic liver disease many years before, on a Christmas morning; she was only twenty-six. Patricia was always honest with me; she told me she would never stop drinking, and that she knew it would kill her. Other drinkers swore tearfully that they would quit, only to relapse within a week of discharge. Patricia was consistent, a true alcoholic; she had the pure, malignant addiction of Nicolas Cage's character in *Leaving Las Vegas*. In the last week of Patricia's life, I stopped all tests, interventions, treatments. Her mother cradled her: a pietà in the observation unit of the ward. When Patricia died, she was both relieved and heartbroken.

The mortuary phoned me to ask if I wanted a post-mortem. 'I'm sorry to call you on Christmas Day when you're not on call,' said the mortician, 'but you know I have to ask, and the juniors on call didn't know the girl, and weren't sure about a post-mortem.'

The first patient at the clinic was a woman with bowel incontinence, who complained bitterly about her plight, showing me a used nappy in a yellow plastic bag. I reminded her that she hadn't turned up for the colonoscopy I had booked for her.

'My daughter puts all the letters in a drawer and forgets them,' she said. Not a convincing excuse, I thought, but I offered to rebook her.

'How long will *that* be? I'm sick of waiting.'

A woman in her late fifties, referred by her GP for 'urgent investigation of profound weight loss'. She told me that she thought her weight loss was caused by 'severe stress'. I asked her about this stress. She hesitated for a moment, and then told her story:

'I've been married for thirty years. Me and my husband lead separate lives. We don't sleep together. We stayed married for the kids. It worked for years. And then the stupidest thing happened. I fell in love with this man I knew from school.

I was like a teenager. His wife found out and he broke it up. I didn't know where I was, or what I was doing. I couldn't eat, I couldn't sleep.'

She composed herself. 'I'm over it now.'

I weighed her; she had regained several kilos since the GP referred her. For the first and last time, I made a formal diagnosis of 'lovesickness'.

The psychotherapist Frank Tallis wrote about lovesickness in his book *The Incurable Romantic: And Other Tales of Madness and Desire* (2018), arguing that modern culture has 'trivialised an important aspect of the human condition and at a very high cost'. Lovesickness, he writes, 'was considered a legitimate diagnosis from classical times to the eighteenth century, but it more or less disappeared in the nineteenth century. Today the term "lovesickness" is employed as a metaphor rather than a diagnosis.' How often over the many years, I wondered, had I missed this diagnosis?

Lovesickness is a kind of grief. I recalled an elderly man who attended my outpatients when I worked in the NHS. His abdominal symptoms were refractory to every treatment I had tried. Finally, at his umpteenth visit, he broke down, weeping.

'What's the matter?' I asked.

'It's my dog. I was too ashamed to tell you. You'd think I was a soppy fool. My dog died and I can't get over it.'

An Indian student with abdominal pain. She showed me pictures on her phone of her stool and told me that she suspected a housemate of poisoning her.

'Why would she do that?'

'She is jealous.'

⟶

At the X-ray conference, Tim – our regular radiologist – was back from holiday, but not noticeably refreshed by the break. His increasing irritability had a comedic zest to it. He struggled to conceal his contempt for over-investigation by us physicians, and cagey, defensive over-reporting by his fellow radiologists. When one of my colleagues asked him, after reviewing countless CT scans, whether this patient should have any 'further imaging', he snapped.

'Is there anything to be said for another mass?'*

The room went quiet.

'Ah sure, why not? Do another fucking scan.'

⟶

When I did my ward round that afternoon, I started with a 'special' patient of a now retired doctor. This man had been admitted acutely over the weekend. He dictated his own treatment, refusing a drug that was clearly indicated. Now he was very ill and needed urgent surgery. He accepted this news without rancour, relieved that someone was finally telling him what had to be done.

---

* This is a famous quote – so famous it's now a meme – from *Father Ted*. Father Dougal is in mortal danger; Ted and two other priests, Father Beeching and Father Clarke, try to brainstorm a solution. They smoke, they scribble ideas on a blackboard; finally, Father Beeching asks: 'Is there anything to be said for another mass?'

*

Sister Walburga died without attempted resuscitation. Colette, the Green Woman, discharged herself over the weekend, but came back; somehow, she found the strength to assault another patient. In a last desperate attempt to rescue her failing liver, we gave her steroids; predictably enough, the steroids did not alleviate her jaundice but *did* give her the worst oral candidiasis (thrush) I had ever seen. This rendered her temporarily speechless.

As I was concluding my round, a manager sped through the ward. She walked on high heels with quick, stabbing steps; always on the phone, taking her instructions directly from Beelzebub.

Tracey

Before I started the ward round, my registrar told me that the 'special' patient had had an emergency operation. I met his surgeon, who estimated his chance of survival at 50 per cent. Had he taken the drug prescribed for him over the weekend, it might not have come to this.

The nurses in the five-day ward* were becoming increasingly agitated by the behaviour of a woman, one of our liver patients, who had come in for the day to have fluid drained from her abdomen (paracentesis). Routine blood tests showed that she was anaemic; the intern told her that she couldn't go home that day as planned, that she would need to stay for a blood transfusion and investigation of this anaemia. She responded to this news by shouting obscenities at the intern and the nurses. When I arrived, she was in a wheelchair, propelling

* A ward open Monday to Friday for patients undergoing elective procedures.

herself along the ward, paddling with her feet. Although we had drained off eight litres of fluid, her belly was still very distended, and her ankles were elephantine. She would be dead within a year, I reasoned, why fret about this anaemia? When I told her she could go, she rose from the wheelchair and hugged me.

A man with a cancerous liver tumour asked me if he could have a drink when he went home. I said yes, that should be fine, thinking if that were me, I would give myself over *entirely* to drink. On the same ward, a young Australian nurse was on the phone to the switchboard: 'I've been trying to get hold of one of Dr Murphy's team for *two hours.*' I envied Dr Murphy for his apparent personal immunity to phone calls from the ward.

Further down the ward, a nurse-manager was ranting at a group of nurses – all of them Indian; they listened to her tirade in complete silence. Although most of the nurses in the ministry were still Irish, many – if not most – of the new jobs were filled by Indians and Filipinos. The young Irish nursing graduates gave their damning verdict on the health service by emigrating to Britain and Australia.

As I saw all the newly qualified doctors on the wards, I recalled the shock of internship – the first job after graduation. The most academically gifted person in my class couldn't bear the messiness, the constant aggression and hostility, the almost complete uselessness of what he had studied so assiduously for six years. After the intern year, he retreated to the laboratory and never again came near the wards.

There was another life in the ministry grounds. The smokers enjoyed their vice in their cars, windows down if the weather permitted. The fitness enthusiasts power-walked or jogged around the perimeter of the grounds. Others lay on the grassy banks, reading or sunbathing. Wild raspberries grew on the fence of the rear car park. The fruit was a deep orange, not the usual pink; nobody ate them.

I went to the shopping centre to buy my mother a birthday present. The woman at the chocolate shop said: 'You don't sound like you're from Cork.' It is vaguely insulting to be accused by a fellow Corkonian of *not* having a Cork accent. I told her that I had grown up less than a mile away. 'You sound more Dublin – educated, like,' she responded in the sing-song local accent. Our conversation was ended by a call from my registrar, who wanted to know what to do about the result of a blood test.

An email from an addiction counsellor about one of our liver patients. Tracey was only twenty-one, but already had full-blown alcoholic cirrhosis; she held the record for the youngest person ever to receive this diagnosis from our service. Tracey had achieved this after a mere seven years of drinking, and without the assistance of hepatitis C. (The combination of alcohol and the hepatitis C virus is particularly toxic to the liver.) She had appeared before the District Court on charges of theft and public disorder. The judge imposed a suspended sentence on condition that Tracey would agree to go to a residential centre for detoxification. Tracey agreed and, after much negotiation, completion of paperwork, and – mysteriously – a *dental* assessment, she was admitted to one such centre. The counsellor wrote:

> I regret to inform you that Tracey was discharged from the detox unit on Sunday. She drank and brought alcohol into the unit on Sunday; she also brought in alcohol for all the residents.
>
> Should Tracey request further treatment for her alcohol dependence, our team will propose an interagency meeting with all care providers together with Tracey and her family.
>
> As yet, we have had no contact with Tracey.

To the eye clinic for another review. I waited for some time. Sam examined me carefully. The detachment was no worse, the retina was intact. What ailed me, he joked, was 'an old man's condition'.

I stayed on for an extraordinary general meeting of the consultants; the chairman of medical staff called this meeting because of 'growing concern' about the lack of consultant representation on the ministry's executive management board. Including me, three showed up. Pretending that I had been called away, I left.

'The *bastards* always do well'

The 'special' patient, whose chance of survival after surgery was estimated at 'fifty-fifty', had improved enough to leave the intensive care unit. 'The *bastards* always do well,' remarked a liver specialist I once worked with. He shared this aperçu while we witnessed the miraculous recovery of a violent criminal. This man had done time in prison for drug dealing and aggravated assault. Following a row with his girlfriend, he had taken a large paracetamol overdose, which caused acute liver failure; he was transferred from his local hospital to the regional liver unit, where he was given a transplant. We speculated on the no doubt blameless and exemplary life of the donor. In the days following the transplant, he was expected to die, having succumbed to infection, kidney failure and graft rejection.* Somehow, he survived, sustained by something we couldn't quite explain – his intrinsic *badness*?

---

* Where the transplanted organ is rejected by the recipient's immune system.

*

A man of sixty-five had come in over the weekend with a large bleed from oesophageal varicose veins, a complication of liver cirrhosis. Even though he drank a minimum of eight pints of stout every day, he was surprised when I told him that he probably had cirrhosis. He thought that only *spirits* could cause this.*

Another newly diagnosed liver cirrhosis patient was also astonished that her nightly naggin† of whiskey could cause such damage. Naturally, she blamed the GP: if he had prescribed a sleeping tablet – as she had pestered him to do – she wouldn't have *needed* to drink a naggin every night to get to sleep.

Gary, yet another liver patient, had been rejected by the detox centre, the same unit that had expelled Tracey. Gary had 'multiple substance issues': dependent on alcohol, methadone,

---

* I have a theory – so far unsullied by evidence – that many people get liver cirrhosis because they don't get hangovers: they are constitutionally immune to them. A hangover, I believe, is an evolutionary protective mechanism to stop us from drinking *quite* so much. I always asked my liver patients about their experience of hangover. Many, particularly the pint drinkers, told me they rarely – or never – got one. One man who continued to drink after the diagnosis of cirrhosis – although, to his credit, he reduced his intake from ten pints a day to four – when asked the hangover question, told me: 'I did *once*. After a wedding.' This wedding has long held a special place in my imagination.

† In Ireland, a naggin is a 200 ml bottle of spirits.

Valium and nicotine. As always, he steered the conversation around to opiates, complaining of 'terrible' back pain.

Colette, the Green Woman, discharged herself as soon as her thrush got better. 'I have a job to do,' she said.

'What's that?' I asked.

'I'd rather not say.'

⌒

Over tea, my registrar told me that he had been on call over the weekend and had presided over the deaths of three very elderly patients, all in their nineties, sent in by ambulance from nursing homes. They were moribund when they arrived, comatose and Cheyne-Stoking; all three died within an hour of arrival in the emergency department. The registrar was so traumatised by this cynical 'turfing'* that he had to be consoled by Dinny the mortician, who gave him tea and toast in the mortuary office.

Over the years, Dinny had comforted many – relatives, doctors, police officers – in this sanctum. When he first came to the ministry in the early 1980s, he was called a mortician; then he became an anatomical pathology technician; now he was mortuary and bereavement services manager. Sometimes, when I had no official reason to visit the mortuary, I called into his office just to hear Dinny talk, to be overwhelmed by

* To get rid of a patient. The phrase was popularised by Samuel Shem's 1978 novel *The House of God*.

the force of his personality, to be reassured that someone as *good* as him was still at the ministry.

Dinny likened his work to running a theatre or an opera house: 'seats, tickets, tea, ice cream'. He deftly handled each professional group – undertakers, social workers, doctors, coroners – like an impresario. Dinny stoically accepted that the bereaved sometimes took out their grief and pain on the institution and its staff. He adapted with equanimity to societal changes: the rise in marital breakdown led to much confusion over who was 'next of kin'; he had seen off several attempts by relatives to sue the ministry for post-traumatic stress disorder after seeing the body of the 'loved one'. The only development he could not reconcile himself to was cremation, which he regarded as 'cruel, unchristian and *English*'.

It was fitting that the dead went to Dinny's tender care. Their suffering was over. He alone rescued the ministry from being a mere charnel house. 'Comfort,' he would say, 'costs nothing.'

I went to the cardiac intensive care unit to consult on a patient; I was there for some time as the intensive care consultant on duty that day liked to discuss cases in elaborate detail. I didn't mind; I had time. The patient was a local; I could see the street where she lived from the unit, which was on the top floor of the cardiac renal building and had the best view in the ministry.

I looked out at the city's western suburbs and pointed out to my registrar the surgeries of the many single-handed

GPs servicing that now ageing population. Most practised in semi-detached suburban houses (often grandly called a 'health centre'), their staff just a secretary, their equipment a prescription pad and a stethoscope. Their elderly clientele was perfectly happy with this, the personal relationship far more important to them than up-to-date technology. How did these doctors manage, working alone? Who did they turn to when they weren't sure what was wrong with a patient? I couldn't imagine this professional isolation. For twenty years, I had regularly – almost daily – knocked on my colleagues' doors, asking: 'Can I pick your brains? What would *you* do with this?'

These were questions that never troubled Harold Shipman.*

---

* In 2000, Dr Harold Shipman, who had practised as a single-handed GP in Hyde near Manchester, was found guilty of the murder of fifteen patients under his care, although the total number of his victims has been estimated to be around 250. He killed his patients by injecting them with diamorphine (heroin). An inquiry chaired by the judge Dame Janet Smith produced a report in 2005, which led to major changes in medical practice in Britain, one of the most significant being the move from single-doctor to multiple-doctor practices.

Shipman graduated from Leeds University medical school in 1970. One of my colleagues when I worked in the NHS was a classmate of his; the class thirty-year reunion dinner in 2000 was cancelled. The medical school, said my colleague, 'didn't want that kind of publicity'. Shipman hanged himself at Wakefield Prison in 2004.

Smoking is good for you

My first clinic patient was a seventy-year-old woman sent by her GP for 'urgent investigation of severe bowel urgency'. She told me that her bowel urgency had resolved after the elimination of gravy and Spanish red wine from her diet. She stressed that her intolerance was to *Spanish* red wine; she could consume all other wines, both red and white, with no ill-effects on her bowels.

A woman in her thirties who had developed multiple unexplained symptoms, which she believed were caused by toxic fumes emanating from a factory near her home. The health and safety authority had investigated her claims and found no basis for them. She was not reassured, suspecting that there had been some kind of 'cover-up'. She had already seen a rheumatologist, a chest physician, a neurologist, a pain specialist and a psychiatrist. She was now on fifteen medications, including two opiates. I asked if she was taking a legal case against this factory: she was. Her patienthood was now so all-consuming that not even a huge financial settlement would cure her.

A woman with colitis, who wouldn't give up her twenty cigarettes a day because it kept her disease in remission; she was probably right.* I came across an old letter in this woman's case notes, dictated in 1984 by Philip, my classmate, friend and fellow intern. Later that year, he moved to London to train as a psychiatrist; this move gave him the freedom to live openly as a gay man. 'Male homosexual acts' were only decriminalised in Ireland in 1993. I never heard from him again.

I did six colonoscopies that afternoon. One young woman enjoyed the sedation rather too much: 'This is *really* good shit,' she drawled. 'What is it?'

*

* Ulcerative colitis is one of a few diseases that smoking protects against. The onset of the disease is sometimes triggered by *giving up* smoking; patients often told me that their disease went into remission when they took up smoking again.

I once attended a session at a conference in the 1990s, the theme of which was 'management of the patient with refractory colitis'. An eminent American gastroenterologist suggested that some patients who did not respond to the standard drugs for colitis should be encouraged to take up 'light smoking'. This assertion was greeted with a collective gasp of horror from the audience, who were outraged that a doctor was *encouraging smoking*.

A woman in her late eighties, sent for colonoscopy by the geriatricians because she had long-standing constipation. I found two tiny polyps.* One of the endoscopy nurses mentioned these polyps to the woman's daughter.

'Why didn't you remove them?' she asked suspiciously. I spent some time explaining the biology and natural history of colonic polyps, and why I had left her elderly mother's polyps alone. She was unconvinced.

Then, the one I had been dreading: Felix. Felix, who was convinced that I was hiding something from him. His colonoscopy was normal: I was wondering how I would break the bad news. He sat in the waiting room drinking tea; a woman of his own age – not his wife – was with him.

'Felix, would you prefer to speak to me on your own?' I asked. He nodded and followed me.

'I don't want payple knowin' me business,' he added, by way of clarification. He took the news surprisingly well and, for the first time, thanked me. I almost skipped back to my office.

⌣⌐

Earlier in the week, I handed over ward duties to a colleague. My registrar informed me that Colette, the Green Woman, had been readmitted, and died the same evening.

---

* The protocols governing colonoscopy mandate the removal of *all* colonic polyps in *all* patients. These protocols were based on three delusions: that resources are limitless, that complications never occur and that people live for ever.

Resentful prisoner

I had seen flashing lights, like falling stars, in my bad eye. Sam warned me to look out for this: it could be a symptom of a retinal detachment. I walked over to the private clinic on the off chance that he might be there. He was, and saw me immediately. No, my retina hadn't detached.

Such access is *the* greatest perk of being a doctor. And this luxury extended to my family. No wonder all those pushy parents want their children to be doctors.

⌁

I was struggling. The arthritis in my hands was getting steadily worse; I ached even after an uneventful endoscopy list, and occasionally got muscle spasms, when I had to put down the scope and wait for it to pass. This vitreous detachment in my eye was not a catastrophe, but it was a signal. I was weary, too, a fatigue that no holiday could reverse.

Medicine is not a good career to grow old in. There is some

truth in the old cliché, 'young doctors and old lawyers'. Surgeons over the age of sixty cause more complications compared to their younger colleagues; older doctors are also more likely to be sued. Physicians (as opposed to surgeons) can compensate to a certain extent for age-related decline by experience and pattern recognition, but become exhausted by the grind of on-call and acute work. The problem is this: you are expected to do the very same job from the day you take up your consultant post at thirty-five to the day you retire at sixty-five. 'You cannot physically do at 58 what you can do at 28,' a disgruntled accident and emergency consultant (aged fifty-eight) told the *British Medical Journal* in 2008. 'If that was the case, Bobby Charlton would still be playing for Manchester United.'

Michael O'Donnell, the late, great doctor-journalist, coined the term 'resentful prisoner syndrome' to describe 'the boredom and a depressing feeling of imprisonment within a career that offered little flexibility and from which the only escape was a distant pension'. In the US, where doctors do not retire with generous state pensions, many continue working into their seventies, or even eighties: 21 per cent of practising American doctors are over sixty-five. In 2012, *The Washington Post* interviewed the geriatrician William Norcross, who assessed the cognitive abilities of older doctors referred by their hospitals or state medical boards. He estimated that 8,000 doctors with full-blown dementia were practising medicine in the US.

All political careers, they say, end in failure. So too with medicine. I cannot recall one doctor who quit at their peak, who left before the juniors started to snigger on the rounds, before the nurses started covering for them. Not one managed, like

Harold Wilson,* to walk out the front door. The doctor in the last year of his or her career: risk-averse, fearful of incident, the main concern to get through the day with the minimum of fuss. Burnt out or just weary? Burnout could now be diagnosed – like so much else – by a tick-box questionnaire. A friend defined it simply as 'spiritual anaemia'.

The sad, illness-stricken retirements of some I had known: the workaholic cardiologist, stunned by the sudden inactivity into a deep and unshakeable melancholy; the sporty paediatrician reduced to a shuffling wreck by Parkinson's disease; the obstetrician's long, unhappy days filled with boredom and whiskey. The geriatrician, a pioneer in the care of people with dementia, who fell victim to his own disease.

A retirement story. On a New Year's Eve in the mid-1990s, I was senior registrar† on call at an NHS teaching hospital. I was

---

* Enoch Powell, wrote the writer and barrister John Mortimer, 'resented Harold Wilson for having given up power voluntarily. He had always admired the emperor Diocletian for doing this very thing, but Harold Wilson, for Enoch Powell, had somehow spoiled or cheapened the great Emperor's gesture.'

† The grade of senior registrar was abolished in the mid-1990s and replaced by 'specialist registrar'. Senior registrars were typically 'junior' doctors with ten or more years' experience; the grade was the final period of 'training' before appointment to a consultant position. Senior registrars were generally highly capable and very experienced, and effectively functioned as junior consultants. When I worked in the NHS in the 1980s and '90s, the great teaching hospitals were run by senior registrars, leaving the consultants free to pursue other interests, such as research, private practice and medical politics.

called by Colin, the medical registrar, which rather surprised me, because Colin was confident – almost too confident – and rarely summoned help.

'I thrombolysed an MI.'*

'And?'

'And now he's paralysed.'

'Do you want me to come in?'

'I think you'd better.'

The patient was a doctor who had retired, just over a week before, on the day before Christmas Eve. When I arrived, he was in the CT scanner. The radiology registrar was animated by the images; he showed Colin and me how the lining of this man's aorta had stripped away – a dissection. Colin had misdiagnosed this as a heart attack and given the worst possible treatment. It was an understandable error: the electrocardiographic (ECG) changes† in aortic dissection and myocardial infarction could be similar. The thrombolytic drug exacerbated the dissection by triggering bleeding. The dissection had extended down to the spinal arteries, which caused the paralysis. I went with him in the ambulance to the regional cardiac surgery centre, where he died later that night. The driver warned me to be careful driving through the rough district near the hospital on the way home: 'If you stop at a traffic lights, make sure your doors are locked.'

Colin and I never again mentioned that evening.

⌣⌐

* Thrombolysis is the administration of a 'clot-busting' drug; MI is myocardial infarction, or heart attack.

† The ECG is a test of the heart's rhythm and electrical activity.

John Lennard-Jones, the eminent London gastroenterologist, died at the age of ninety-two. His obituary stated the cause of death as 'old age'. He died two weeks after his wife: 'a broken heart' could have been entered in the death certificate as a 'contributing factor'.

Lennard-Jones once visited, in the early 1990s, the unit in Edinburgh where I was a trainee. 'L-J' was a modest, abstemious man, and a devout Christian – some called him 'saintly'. I presume that is why he never became *Sir* John – too nice. My professor gave a dinner in his honour at her home. As the evening wore on, much drink was consumed; a passionate argument broke out, there might have been singing. I recall L-J being unimpressed; had he not been staying the night, he would have left.

'Like a greasy dog'

The first outpatient was a woman in her late twenties who came into the clinic room with her mother. She had that moon face often seen in young female alcoholics.* The mother asked her daughter if she wanted her to stay; she said no, she would prefer to see me alone. I told her that her blood tests showed swelling of her red blood cells – macrocytosis – which strongly suggested that she was drinking too much. She readily agreed and added that her mother too had a problem with alcohol.

A girl of twenty with irritable bowel syndrome. Her GP had written requesting a routine appointment, and then wrote again, asking for this to be upgraded to 'urgent' because she was missing time from her course – 'canine studies, which she loves'. Would this GP have viewed her case as being less

---

* All those late-Stuart-period court beauties painted by Godfrey Kneller had that look; was it because Queen Anne made round faces fashionable, or were they all drinkers?

urgent if she did not 'love' her course, or if the course had been something less worthy than *canine studies*?

A jolly woman in her seventies with abdominal pain. A masseuse told her that she had 'a twisted bowel'.

'She must have marvellously sensitive hands,' I said.

'She's a trainee.'

'Then she has a great future.'

Nikki, a woman of forty, said her chronic constipation was causing headache, dizziness, double vision and 'brain fog'. Her faeces, she told me, smelled 'like a greasy dog'. Many of my patients mysteriously believed that shit and farts should not have an unpleasant odour, that they should be neutral, even pleasant.* 'I am intoxicated,' Nikki said, 'by my own excrement.'

*

* This might be due to the baleful influence of Gillian McKeith, the TV nutritionist: 'The perfect poo should not smell putrid, and it should be a nice conker-brown colour. Foul-smelling stools are a sign of poor digestion and food stagnating in your large intestine. This means you are toxic and your gut is overly acidic. You are sorely in need of digestive enzymes.'

In his *Guardian* 'Bad Science' column, Ben Goldacre raised doubts about McKeith's title of 'doctor'. Her PhD is from the Clayton College of Natural Health, a non-accredited correspondence course college. She is also a certified member of the American Association of Nutritional Consultants; Goldacre purchased a membership on behalf of his dead cat, Hettie, for $60. 'I have the certificate hanging in my loo,' he wrote.

An elderly man with a Liverpudlian accent. He was born there and came to Ireland aged ten in 1950. The Christian brothers in his new school threatened to 'beat that horrible accent' out of him. He held on to it as an act of defiance. Two years ago, he found his daughter dead on the sofa, the TV still on. A brain aneurysm had burst; she died immediately.

⌒

I went, yet again, to the eye clinic.

When Sam finally saw me, it was after seven o'clock, and he still had more patients to see. How little we knew of other departments in the ministry: we all thought that *we* were so busy. My eye was no worse: my vitreous jelly was now floating around in a sea of serous fluid, but the retina was intact.

The seven sins of medicine

My first patient at that morning's clinic was Maddalena, a teenager who was attending several clinics, including rheumatology, neurology, the child and adolescent mental health services, dermatology, the pain service, physiotherapy and dietetics. The paediatricians passed her on to me the minute she reached sixteen; their relief was palpable. Maddalena had multiple symptoms, including blackouts, fatigue, rashes visible only to her parents, chronic limb pain, poor concentration and mood swings, abdominal pain and diarrhoea. When I called her from the waiting room, Maddalena – although taller than me and weighing 76 kg (nearly 12 stone) – was sitting with her head in her father's lap, like a baby.

Attending to Maddalena's many undiagnosed complaints was her Italian father's full-time work. Although scrupulously polite, he had a knack of bullying doctors into doing his bidding, which was generally to send Maddalena for new tests, refer her to other services, and prescribe more medication. Exhausted by his persistence, and mindful of the waiting room full of patients still to see, they usually gave in.

He showed me photos on his phone of Maddalena's stool and asked whether I thought it looked 'inflamed'. Maddalena stared at the floor throughout. When I tried to draw her out by directing questions to her, her father immediately cut in and answered on her behalf. Later that day, I phoned the child and adolescent mental health unit; they told me that Maddalena's psychiatrist had retired, but they would ask the new temporary (locum) consultant to phone me.

All this made me think of Munchausen's syndrome, and Richard Asher (1912–69), who named the condition. Munchausen's syndrome is a 'factitious' disorder: those affected feign illness, in a very extreme form of attention-seeking. In his original 1951 paper in *The Lancet*, Asher gave a colourful account of three patients who went from hospital to hospital in London with dramatic stories, usually of severe abdominal pain and vomiting blood. Asher named the syndrome after the titular hero of Rudolf Erich Raspe's novel *Singular Travels, Campaigns and Adventures of Baron Munchausen* (1781). Raspe's Baron was loosely based on a minor German aristocrat who was notorious for the tall tales he told about his military career in the Russo-Turkish War of 1735–9. 'The persons affected,' wrote Asher, 'have always travelled widely; and their stories, like those attributed to him, are both dramatic and untruthful. Accordingly, the syndrome is respectfully dedicated to the baron, and named after him.' Asher might have been disappointed to learn that the new formulation 'factitious disorder imposed on self' is now preferred.

Munchausen's syndrome *by proxy** is where a parent presents a child with factitious symptoms, and the preferred formulation now for this is 'factitious disorder imposed on *another*'. For a doctor to accuse a parent of Munchausen's syndrome by proxy required both courage and *absolute* certainty: if there was even the remotest possibility of another diagnosis, this allegation could have catastrophic consequences. I recalled a case I had heard of – during my NHS days – about a paediatrician based in the hospital I then worked at, who had made this accusation, only for the child to be diagnosed later with a rare type of spinal tumour.

I didn't think that Maddalena was truly an example of this: the cases I had read about were in much younger children; the parents (nearly always the mother) had often inflicted unspeakable cruelties, including poisoning; Maddalena was just too *healthy*. But there was something about her father's involvement that I could only call *unwholesome*; he did not directly *cause* all these symptoms, but he was gaining, in some way that I couldn't yet figure out, from his daughter's transformation from child to full-time patient. And *she* gave the distinct and unignorable impression of something suppressed, hidden. Her demeanour and posture conveyed one word: *beaten*.

---

* The term Munchausen's syndrome by proxy was coined by the Leeds-based paediatrician Sir Roy Meadow in 1977. Meadow was later disgraced after his testimony as an expert witness contributed to the wrongful conviction of several women (most famously Sally Clark) accused of killing their own children. 'Meadow's Law' (one sudden infant death is a tragedy, two is suspicious, and three is murder) has since been discredited.

*

I came across Asher's collected essays, *Talking Sense*, when I was a medical student; he wrote elegantly and had a refreshingly jaundiced view of his profession. But what drew me back to that frayed yellow paperback was the sense that he was writing through the years directly to *me*. I reread the book with as much pleasure as when I had first greedily consumed it in one sitting.

Although he ran the 'mental observation unit' at the Central Middlesex Hospital in London, Asher loathed psychiatry, which he thought was closer to religion than medicine. In 1964, the hospital authorities appointed a psychiatrist to take charge of this unit; Asher was so offended he resigned. A contemporary at the Central Middlesex later wrote about Asher's 'cyclothymic temperament' and attributed this hasty resignation to 'pique'. He fell into a deep depression and, at fifty-seven, killed himself. *Talking Sense* was published posthumously in 1971; Asher committed suicide in 1969 – barbiturates, I think. Much easier to kill yourself then: a combination of alcohol and barbiturates was highly effective. The 'barbs' were phased out in the 1970s, replaced by the benzodiazepines (Valium and so on). It is almost impossible to kill yourself with 'benzos'; I cannot recall a single fatal overdose.

Asher wrote an essay for *The Lancet* in 1949 called 'The seven sins of medicine', which he listed as: obscurity, cruelty, bad manners, over-specialisation, love of the rare, common stupidity and sloth. There is a brilliant word, by the way, for love of the rare: 'spanophilia' (I had a bad case of this when I first read Asher's essays). I whiled away the wait at the eye clinic by coming up with my own seven deadly sins: venality, humbug, cowardice, neophilia,* Phariseeism, boosterism and sentimentality.

In January 2015, I happened to be in London and went to see an exhibition at the Royal Society of Medicine called 'Richard Asher: a celebration'. The man at reception told me I must be mistaken, there was no such exhibition. 'I've travelled all the way from Ireland just for this,' I lied. 'Can you ask somebody?' He said OK, he would make a phone call. 'No,' he said, 'whatever you're looking for isn't here.' 'Please,' I said, 'I *know* it's on.' He frowned, went off for ten minutes, eventually returned, and grudgingly admitted me to the Society's library, where I spent a happy, solitary hour looking at Asher's papers and letters. The Munchausen man, who once lived on the same street (Wimpole Street) as this august society, was as forgotten as Ozymandias.

John Lennard-Jones was Richard Asher's registrar in the late 1950s; I wish I had known this when I met 'L-J' at that boozy dinner in Edinburgh thirty years ago. He and Asher wrote a paper for *The Lancet* in 1959 called 'Why do they do it? A Study of Pseudocide'. I don't know why they chose the word 'pseudocide', which means a *faked* death, when they were writing about people who self-harmed without wishing to die: 'We call their performance "pseudocide" – a monstrous word which we would gladly relinquish if we knew as good a current one.' I suspect Asher, rather than Lennard-Jones, wrote the text:

* Love of the new or the novel.

Case 5. – An aggressive unlikeable man aged forty-two took to drink, bringing noise and violence to his home.

Case 6. – A man faced with an intolerable situation needed a short holiday in oblivion.

Such attempts ... may occur in children at loggerheads with their parents, in parents who feel neglected by their children in unhappy marriages, and in hot-blooded young men who, in Damon Runyan's inimitable phrase, have 'the big burnt-up feeling that a guy gets when his doll walks out on him'.

No. It must have been Asher; I can't imagine L-J summoning the spirit of Damon Runyan.

A locum consultant from the child and adolescent mental health unit phoned me about Maddalena. I told him that I was worried about her. He hadn't personally seen her, he told me, but he had spoken to one of the nurses there about Maddalena, and no, they were not *especially* worried about her. They would, however, see her again at their clinic. When I put the phone down, I wondered what I should do. How could I possibly help this girl when the psychiatrists were not *especially* worried about her?

My wife and I went for a swim at Dunworley beach, stopping in Timoleague on the way home to buy a newspaper. A woman knocked at the car window; I rolled it down. 'I'm Tommy Murphy's wife!' she said, pointing at her husband – a long-standing patient, who was sitting in his car, smiling and waving. Mrs Murphy addressed my wife: 'Is it true he's retiring?'

Did my patients know something I didn't?

Shit transplant

I saw a woman on the ward, a patient of one of my gastro-enterology colleagues who asked me to give a second opinion. She had a severe, complicated intestinal disease, and had been in hospital for three months. Not surprisingly, she was fed up. The liaison psychiatrist gave this a label of 'adjustment reaction'.

I looked around the ward: the saintly, long-serving clinical nurse manager in deep conversation with a relative; a team of three junior doctors striding down the corridor, with that loud, self-regarding busyness. The nurses and junior doctors worked away quite independently, oblivious of one another, as if they were engaged in diametrically opposed pursuits, independent agencies who just happened to share a workspace.

My first outpatient was Marie, a woman with chronic abdominal pain. She had hired a medium, who came to her house and summoned up two spirits: her cousin (who had died aged thirty in a car crash) and her mother-in-law. Both spirits told Marie that the pain would leave her body, banished like some minor demon.

A frail old man was sent by another service for investigation of anaemia; he could barely walk and had mild dementia. His anaemia was not of the kind that required the attentions of a gastroenterologist, but here he was, a box ticked. By chance, he had developed severe diarrhoea two days before; I guessed this might be caused by infection and started him on an antibiotic. I sent off a stool sample, which later confirmed infection with *clostridium difficile*.* His referral to me was unnecessary, but at least his visit wasn't wasted.

Fionnuala, a young woman with colitis, came for a follow-up appointment. She had been an inpatient a couple of months before; I was then 'on' for the wards, but had to go off sick. I came down with influenza and felt so ill that I went home to bed and switched off my phone. This was only the second time in my career I had ever done so. It was a Friday afternoon, and my last instruction to my registrar was that Fionnuala should be kept in over the weekend. She had a complicated, difficult disease, and I wanted her to stay put until she was in full remission. The bed crisis was even worse than usual

---

* *Clostridium difficile* is a toxin-producing bacterium that is a common cause of acute diarrhoea, particularly in the elderly. Most patients have a history of recent antibiotic exposure.

that day; the nurse manager and clinical director both tried to contact me to ask me to discharge Fionnuala, but I was asleep, my phone switched off. They tried the physician on call, who, having no knowledge of the patient, declined to discharge her. Another consultant who had been involved in her care was persuaded to discharge Fionnuala. I learned about all this only a week later, when I returned to work.

'I'm sorry, Fionnuala,' I said. 'I had no idea.'

'It doesn't matter now,' she said.

I stayed, with no great enthusiasm, for our department's journal club. This educational activity had long been sponsored by the drug reps, who supplied coffee and muffins. This modest investment bought them access to the doctors; some reps were bolder and gave a formal presentation on their product. Doctors' attention is *very* cheaply purchased. The club was meant to give the junior doctors some experience in presenting a summary and critique of important studies published in the medical journals. They were ideally meant to talk a little about the background to the paper, to indicate why it was relevant to clinical practice, and to identify any weaknesses in the work. The trainees who presented at this meeting were usually poorly prepared and uncritical, believing that *anything* published in a medical journal must be true, and read out these papers verbatim. There was nearly always a problem with the computer and the projector. It was regarded as bad form to criticise the juniors' presentations; it might be construed as bullying. Sheila Sherlock would be dismayed by such cowardice.

The drug rep eyed me with malice; she knew my views on 'industry support' for this meeting and regarded my refusal to see reps as shameful, a dereliction of my professional duty. Our house officer presented a paper on faecal transplantation.* This aesthetically unappealing treatment worked well for severe, refractory infection with *clostridium difficile*; now it was being touted as a treatment for colitis, Crohn's disease, irritable bowel syndrome, multiple sclerosis, cancer, obesity, diabetes and *autism*. Why worry about the likes of Gillian McKeith when mainstream 'scientific' medicine makes such claims?

An email to all users:

> Due to unprecedented pressure on hospital capacity the decision has been made to **cancel all elective activity** tomorrow.

'Unprecedented', I thought, means something that has never happened, 'never done or known before', but this kind of 'pressure' was a regular, even frequent, occurrence. The ministry's inadequate bed capacity had been reconfigured, *renarrativised*, as an arbitrary act of a capricious God, an 'unprecedented' event.

---

* Faecal microbiota transplantation (FMT), or 'shit transplant', is the transfer of faeces from a healthy donor to the bowel of the recipient by enema, capsule or colonoscopy.

A letter from the hospice, informing me of the death of a patient of mine with lung cancer. By the time he came to me, his cancer had spread to his bones, liver and brain. The palliative care registrar wrote: 'He had full insight into his condition and spoke about not wanting chemotherapy due to the potential side effects. He expressed some concern that he would be committing suicide if he refused treatment, we reassured him that this was not the case.'

That afternoon, I happened to be in this hospice to visit a relative. As I drove in, I pulled up next to a former classmate, a surgeon whose cancer was now advanced. He was attending the hospice now as a day patient for 'symptom control'. We were not friends, but we were *friendly*. 'How are things?' I asked. 'So-so,' he replied in a weak, reedy voice, and drove off.

Maurice

All the important people deserted the hospital in August. To be seen in the ministry during this month was an admission of failure: you *should* be in your summer house in west Cork. The first Monday in September saw the return of the important people and the medical students. It was the official first day of the season. I was not surprised, therefore, to find Maurice, striding along the main corridor, with that burnished, stylish tan you get only from sailing.

Some years ago, while still in his early forties, Maurice had grown weary of clinical work. He knew he had to escape, but only in a respectable way, a way that would allow him to maintain his income and continue to enjoy the prestige of the profession. He steadily built a portfolio of roles for himself outside the ministry, attaching himself to various educational, training and regulatory bodies. He became an advisor – a 'key opinion leader' – to three drug companies and was appointed to the boards of two health quangos. Maurice eventually accrued so many of these roles that he was able to put in place a complex financial arrangement whereby his clinical 'sessions' were 'bought out' using money given to the ministry by a number of these external bodies. This paid for a succession of locum doctors who did his clinical work, so Maurice could be 'freed up' to pursue his activities on behalf of these bodies. As the years went by, the trail leading to this money – or more correctly, *monies* – became so overgrown that not even Maurice was quite sure who was still paying, and how much. He was reassured: if *he* did not know, then it was highly improbable that some nosy manager would cause him any trouble. All he knew was that the ministry continued to employ the locums, and he continued to receive his full salary. The locums generally stayed for less than a year, but Maurice was assiduous in identifying replacements, so his neglected service bumbled along somehow. He was caught out just once, when he had to look after the wards for an entire month.

Maurice was careful with his sinecure: he maintained a foothold in the hospital – a monthly clinic, which happened to be today. This clinic was not a great burden for Maurice: he allowed a maximum of ten follow-up bookings and insisted that two registrars be present to assist him; it was, he said, 'a great educational opportunity for them'. This undemanding commitment allowed Maurice to talk gravely about 'the intense pressure we front-line clinicians face'. He opined about this so often that he eventually began to believe what he was saying: this added an unexpected touch of authenticity to his pronouncements. He could believe two opposing truths; it was a useful attribute, like being ambidextrous. He spoke solemnly at graduation ceremonies about the privilege of practising medicine. In his many radio and television interviews he always alluded to his clinical work: 'When I visited the emergency department yesterday...' At academic gatherings, research conferences and committee meetings, he would solemnly state: 'I am first and foremost a clinician.' Maurice successively presented himself as a champion of patients with a rare disease, as a pioneer of digital health, and as a spokesman for 'the coalface clinicians'.

He had a Widmerpoolian talent for being on the cusp of – and usually ahead of – any new trend. He tweeted, he blogged, he podcasted. He was an enthusiastic early adopter of new protocols, new diseases, new ways of communicating. He was 'passionate', he said, about mandatory open disclosure of medical error, knowing that *he* would never have to disclose anything, since he did virtually no clinical work. He was passionate about many things, including patient-centred care, partnership with pharmaceutical companies, and 'disruptive' technologies.

Maurice travelled for much of the year, representing these various bodies in the Far East and North America. He was away so often that one wag, encountering him in the ministry on a Friday afternoon, asked him if the airport was closed. He had so many affiliations that none of his many offices and bases could be sure at any one time where exactly Maurice was. This gave him great manoeuvrability.

Maurice maintained a private practice, seeing only patients suffering from a condition that was bothersome enough for them to seek his expertise, but which had never been known to kill anyone. He was a good listener and talked sympathetically to patients about food intolerance and microbial imbalances. Private practice, he said, kept him 'clinically sharp'. Maurice had a reputation among this patient community for being 'open to new ideas'.

Maurice was envied by his colleagues because he had maximised the rewards of the profession, while minimising – indeed, eliminating – the burdensome obligations. He had found the sweet spot where free-riding* could be maximised without sacrificing status, prestige or income. His was the quintessentially successful medical career of the twenty-first century.

Maurice stopped and warmly asked after my family.

---

* In his 2005 paper 'Personal view: passing the buck and taking a free ride – a game-theoretic approach to evasive management strategies in gastroenterology', the American physician Amnon Sonnenberg wrote:

'Free-riding physicians enjoy the status, prestige and income without fully contributing to its overall mission. By shifting the costs of potential medical complications and difficult patient encounters to other physicians, they reap the benefits of their profession without carrying its full weight.

'From a physician's perspective, the management of a given medical problem is associated with benefits, as well as costs. The benefits include a sense of accomplishment, patient satisfaction and gratitude, self-respect and professional fulfilment, professional reputation, continued employment and financial compensation. The costs include the amount of time spent on a medical case, mental and physical workload, fear of failure, humiliation, harassment by patient and family, tainted professional record and possible litigation. The interactions between any two physicians can be formulated in terms of a non-zero-sum game between two adversaries.

'Within a small group of coworkers, a free rider would eventually compromise her professional reputation and become shunned by other members of the group. In contradistinction, the administrative structures of large medical centers with many encounters among anonymous health care providers are more prone to breed such tendencies.'

A long lie

An elderly couple were the first to arrive at that morning's outpatients. When I saw his wife in the waiting room, in a wheelchair, I assumed that *she* was the patient, but no, it was *him* – 'she goes everywhere with me'. *He* had had abdominal pain on and off for fifteen years. I reassured him that 'anything serious would have declared itself by now'.

'They said the same thing to my mother.'

'What happened to her?'

'She died of cancer.'

'What age was she?'

'Ninety.'

Next, a young woman who talked at length about her food intolerances, which caused bloating, headache, fatigue, backache. She could eat *turkey*, she said, but not *chicken*; she could manage *pasta*, but not *bread*. She had an expression of infinite suffering, borne bravely.

Much of my time at the outpatient clinic was spent

discussing food intolerances and allergies. I told all my patients that *intolerance* and *allergy* were quite different,* and that the only two food intolerances I could reliably diagnose were coeliac disease (caused by gluten sensitivity) and lactose intolerance. Most of my patients with irritable bowel syndrome much preferred food intolerance to 'stress' as an explanation for their symptoms. They saw food as full of potential dangers, an alien invader of their defenceless bodies. This belief was driven by freely available misinformation from a variety of media. There was something comforting for them, I think, about this belief: what was ailing them came from *outside*. To admit to 'stress' was to admit to weakness, to human frailty; to suffer from food intolerance was to be a blameless victim of a malign external force. With a few, this obsession was an expression of vanity and solipsism. And one should never underestimate the power of modishness: gluten always topped the list of suspects, but its pre-eminence was increasingly threatened by upstart challengers, such as 'carbs', 'dairy', caffeine and 'FODMAPs'.†

---

* An allergic reaction to food usually occurs immediately, typically with a rash or wheezing. True allergy is an immune reaction and is uncommon. Offending foods (such as peanuts and shellfish) can be identified by blood or skin-prick tests. Intolerance is much vaguer; it is not an acute immune reaction, and the symptoms are generally mild and vague. Many would argue that the term 'intolerance' has little or no scientific basis, a catch-all term for any reaction to food – real or imaginary – that does not have an immune basis. Surveys of the adult population in the UK reported that 20 to 30 per cent believe they have a food allergy or intolerance.

† 'FODMAP' is an acronym for Fermentable Oligo-, Di-, Mono-saccharides And Polyols. These are types of sugars, present in various fruits and vegetables, which are broken down ('fermented') by bacteria in the gut, producing gas, which can cause bloating, farting and discomfort. The more enterprising food stores now have 'FODMAP-free' sections.

The trick to doing this outpatient clinic was to *not switch off* during these long discussions about food intolerance; the next patient might well have a serious disease. Gastroenterology is a strange speciality; I spent half the day on the wards attending my often moribund liver disease patients, and the other half in the outpatients listening to people who thought they might be allergic to *wheat*, but not *gluten*?

I did my round in the afternoon, seeing twenty patients in ten wards. A seventy-eight-year-old woman, now in the fiftieth day of her stay, had spent the first week in the intensive care unit with sepsis (caused by a urinary infection) and delirium. Now, several weeks on, she was still raving mad. Her family, I was told, wanted 'maximum intervention'.

An alcoholic woman in her sixties, with the fruity accent of the city's professional class – on first-name terms with nearly every doctor and lawyer in Cork – told me she was 'temporarily' living in a nursing home.

A man in his seventies had been admitted after a fall. He lived alone and was on the ground for several hours – a 'long lie' – before a neighbour found him and called an ambulance. His muscle had broken down, releasing into his bloodstream a protein called myoglobin, which caused transient kidney failure. He was on dialysis for a few days; his kidneys recovered.

I recognised him immediately: I had seen him nearly twenty years before when he returned from a holiday with jaundice. This was caused by hepatitis B, which he had acquired in an Amsterdam brothel.

'I've seen you before,' I said.

'In what context?' he asked suspiciously.

'In this hospital. You as a patient, me as your doctor.'

'I don't think so,' he snorted.

An eighty-year-old woman with lung cancer. She had gone with chest pain to a private hospital two months before and was found to have fluid around her lung. They sent her to the ministry's thoracic surgery unit for a biopsy. The chest surgeons found a large malignant mass with secondary deposits in her ribs and spine. She had several sessions of 'palliative' radiation treatment; the oncologists advised against chemotherapy. She came back into the ministry with a chest infection, and was admitted under our service, which happened to be on call that day for general medicine. Now she was drowsy and in pain; she was being fed through a nasogastric tube and was on intravenous antibiotics. The palliative care doctors said her pain control was 'difficult', that the opiates were too strong for her.

'How much does she know?' I asked my registrar.

'Not a lot.'

Had anyone had the difficult conversation with her? Probably not. Whose responsibility was it? The consultant in the private hospital? The chest surgeons? The radiation specialists? The oncologists? The palliative care physicians? Me? *Now* was not a good time, I thought; she was too drowsy and in too much pain. And what was the point of the nasogastric feeding and the antibiotics? I thought of stopping both, but I had not met the family yet; what if they were the 'so you're just going to let Mum die' type? The tube-feeding had been instigated by the dieticians, who were concerned that this dying woman was not meeting her 'nutritional targets'. Weight loss in people with cancer was now called sarcopenia;* something to be investigated, quantified, intensively treated.

So easy to *start* treatments, so difficult to stop. Everyone involved treated this woman correctly and by protocol; collectively, we had inflicted only suffering.

⌒

'The only means to truly reduce adverse events is to avoid patient encounters altogether.' (Amnon Sonnenberg, 'Adverse outcomes: why bad things happen to good people', *Clinical Gastroenterology and Hepatology*, 2015.)

---

* Sarcopenia, literally 'lack of flesh'. The word was first used to describe the muscle loss that occurs normally with ageing. Now that ageing has been reconfigured as a 'disease', so too has sarcopenia. This 'condition' has its own journals, conferences and experts; much of this academic activity is sponsored by companies that manufacture expensive nutritional 'supplements'.

Dr Jack's 'Rap R'

A newspaper headline quoted the president of the Irish Hospital Consultants Association, who predicted that 2019/20 will be 'the worst ever winter trolley crisis'. I found these apocalyptic predictions strangely and inexplicably comforting. When I arrived at the ministry in 2001, I was appalled that patients who were admitted to hospital through the emergency department were often accommodated on a trolley in the corridor. I had never seen this in my many years working in the NHS. This daily outrage against human dignity was tacitly accepted by the Irish. Every winter, it would get slightly worse, and every winter, the Irish news and current affairs television programme *Prime Time* would do a hand-wringing 'special' on the trolley crisis, featuring a different, furrow-browed minister for health promising that improvements were underway. The Irish nurses and midwives' organisation kept a daily tally of the 'trolley count', as did the Irish Health Service Executive; these counts were often at variance, which sometimes triggered ill-tempered spats.

For the patients, it was undignified and intolerable. For the doctors, like me, who saw most of their newly admitted patients in these circumstances, it was an abandonment of professional standards we held dear. The heart of clinical medicine is the history and physical examination; it was difficult to take a history from a frail elderly person with poor hearing who was lying on a trolley in the corridor of the emergency department, and to examine them properly was almost impossible. This first encounter with the patient was the most important, and already your work as a doctor was substandard and compromised.

My registrar phoned to tell me that the well-connected alcoholic woman (the one who knew every lawyer and doctor in Cork) was in a rage, demanding to be discharged. She was being detained against her will, she said, and would call the police. She wasn't yet ready for discharge, needing several more days of intravenous antibiotics for her chest infection. Luckily, the clinical nurse manager in charge of that ward was the most capable in the ministry and had organised everything (ambulance transport, nursing home) by the time I arrived. All I had to do was to get my patient to sign the form confirming that she was 'self-discharging against medical advice'. Sweaty, pop-eyed and red-faced, she contemptuously scratched something illegible and threw the paper back at me.

Dealing with such incidents, I reflected, required the skills of a policeman, or a pub landlord, rather than those of a physician. I wondered, too, why the registrar thought this was a task that required *my* involvement. And I mused that all the time I had devoted as a trainee to research might have been more usefully spent shadowing a nightclub bouncer or a warder in a high-security prison. Not once have I ever thought, yes, the three years I spent in an Edinburgh laboratory researching mucosal immunology *really* helped on the wards today, yet every day I was talking down angry drunks, calming delirious old folk, defusing the wrath of 'difficult' families.

⌣⁀

The grand round* was the ministry's showcase academic

* Grand rounds probably began in the late nineteenth century at Johns Hopkins medical school during William Osler's tenure as professor of medicine (1889–1905). The rounds were traditionally organised by the residents (trainee doctors) and were described by the editor of the *New England Journal of Medicine* Franz Ingelfinger as 'decorous, stately and punctual'. Patients were usually brought to the lecture theatre and were often questioned or examined by senior doctors.

The grand round (also held on Wednesdays) at the Royal Postgraduate Medical School at London's Hammersmith Hospital was a celebrated institution of British medicine during its golden age when Sir John McMichael and Sheila Sherlock were in their pomp. The junior doctors who presented were generally terrified, so aggressive was the questioning by the senior staff. The late Graham Neale, who worked there in the 1960s and '70s, wrote in 1989: 'It [the Hammersmith grand round] remains without equal because, as from the beginning, every consultant physician attends; because the centrepiece is the patient who is presented in person; and because the junior staff present data which show their ability to observe and to investigate as if the patient's illness was designed to help further our knowledge of disease... The end result is a debate which is testing for junior staff, usually exciting and often heated, but never intentionally unkind.'

It is rare now for patients to be 'shown' at these gatherings, which have gradually lost their prestige and importance to the life of a hospital. I cannot recall a single instance of a patient being the centre of the event, held in the main lecture theatre (which accommodated over 200) over lunch hour on Wednesdays. This week's grand round could not have been more prescient: 'Mastering effective communication', presented by a visiting English speaker known to all as 'Dr Jack'. He had worked as a psychiatrist for many years but became bored and gave it up at forty. He could afford to do so; he had inherited wealth. At a loss for something to do, he had a Pauline conviction that he should set up a communication skills training company. Although he had no special aptitude for this – he was not renowned as a great speaker – Dr Jack was a blank canvas on which all new fads and fashions could be projected. He prepared himself by attending workshops at Harvard Medical School; he borrowed the catchiest phrases and most modish ideas and made them his own. 'Rap R' was established, with Dr Jack as chief executive.

Dr Jack's only client was the British state, but this client was a voracious purchaser of his services. He ran workshops for doctors, for nurses, for therapists of all denominations, for anyone working in health care. Those attending dozed through the sessions, content that their employer was paying, and that they had fulfilled their mandatory requirement for 'continuing professional development'. Dr Jack was popular because he always finished the workshops early: 'I know you all have trains to catch.'

He collaborated with famous sportspersons, whose recycled pep talks on 'leadership', 'teamwork' and 'resilience' could be

---

ministry's grand round. 'Grand rounds are not so grand anymore,' lamented Lawrence Altman in *The New York Times* in 2006. The Oslerian ideal has given way to dense PowerPoint presentations, as prestige within medicine seeped from the bedside to the research laboratory.

applied to almost any human endeavour.* Those attending his courses got a vicarious thrill from meeting these heroes, and proudly shared with friends and families what the famous rugby player had told them over coffee.

Dr Jack's grand round talk was composed entirely of phrases like 'co-facilitation', 'mentalisation' and 'reflective space'. No phrase was too hackneyed or clichéd for him to employ, no whimsical cartoon too forced or too twee for him to illustrate his concepts with. He had invented catchy acronyms, such as 'HELP', 'TALK', 'HEAR', which were illustrated with huge PowerPoint ziggurats. Throughout this talk, Dr Jack maintained a forced, rather sinister rictus. He made frequent mention of his experience in psychiatry, an occupation he had abandoned with little regret. Towards the end, he showed an animated cartoon, featuring anthropomorphised animals, to illustrate what empathy was. He paused theatrically and declared: 'If I could use one word to explain what I do, and *why* I do it, that word would be *empathy*.'

* In 2001, I found myself in a Barcelona hotel listening to such a talk by the athlete Kriss Akabusi, who gave a manic motivational speech, frequently enlivened by his 'famous laugh'. I couldn't bear it, and left after five minutes, much to the chagrin of the drug reps who had hired Akabusi.

'They'll bugger off elsewhere'

I started the round on my home ward. The first patient was an angry woman; she was angry because no doctor would be the captain of her ship. She had complex bowel and liver problems, for which she had undergone several operations. She had been admitted with sepsis on six occasions over eight months, in two hospitals under several consultants.

A tiny, bird-like woman had been treated successfully for fluid retention in her abdomen,* but expressed great reluctance to leave. She liked it here on the ward, she told me; there was always company, and the nurses were nice to her. This crowded, noisy ward was, for this woman, better than home.

A man who had been an inpatient for several weeks had many problems, but the main one now was a contracture of his right

* Ascites, usually caused by liver cirrhosis.

103

knee. The orthopaedic surgeons put on a plaster-of-Paris cast; the physiotherapist complained that the cast was not straight enough and would not correct the contracture. The orthopaedic service, predictably, declined to take over this man's care, so a gastroenterologist (me) was now peering at his bent knee and unsuitable cast. The physiotherapist did not conceal her opinion of my expertise in the management of contractures.

A super-tanker patient – my colleague's – scuttled down the ward, a bag of liquid feed on a drip stand, propelled by little wheels. A very grand senior physician* in my NHS days – so grand, he was known as 'the Duke' – once advised me that the best way of getting rid of super-tankers and heart-sinks was to deliberately quarrel with them: 'They'll bugger off elsewhere,' he said cheerfully. You might have got away with this in the 1980s; now, it would be likely to backfire.

The woman with lung cancer – who had been moved on by so many services – had gone to the hospice; perhaps the difficult conversation will happen there. Or perhaps not.

Mr Jones, a man admitted two months before, following a fall – which fractured his pelvis – had never recovered and was now dying in a side room on the cardiac ward. The main concern

---

* Handsome in a jowly way, with just a hint of raised eyebrow. Geoffrey Palmer would have been perfect casting.

was whether the coroner should be informed when he died: any death related to trauma had to be referred. This man was dying, not because of the fracture, but because he was too old and frail to get better; he simply had nothing left.

Walking through the stroke ward, I met the daughter of a friend, now an intern, the lowest rank of junior doctor. She had qualified as a barrister, and here she was, clerking new patients and putting in drips, but seemed happy enough. Why did so many doctors' children become doctors themselves? A GP friend told me that his son was inspired to follow him when he witnessed his father resuscitating a choking man in a café. This uplifting tale might have been more plausible had this son gone on to become, say, an intensivist, but no, he was training in *psychiatry*. Doctors like these stories, these foundation myths of their vocation: 'and that's when I decided to be a doctor.'

When I was a student, I knew a man called John Bradshaw (1918–89). He qualified as a doctor in Liverpool, but early in his career became disenchanted with medicine and gave it up for writing. In 1978 he wrote *Doctors on Trial*, a polemic against modern medicine, very much influenced by Ivan Illich.* His son told me many years after his death that Bradshaw, despite his jeremiad against medicine, was 'extremely disappointed' that none of his children had become a doctor.

* Ivan Illich (1926–2002), the Austrian priest, philosopher and social critic, author of *Medical Nemesis* (1975).

Many of those who worked in the ministry were related: not just the doctors, but *everyone* – nurses, porters, cleaners, security personnel, secretaries, clerks. After forty years, some were third-generation ministry people. The medical students and junior doctors attached to my unit were very often the children of my colleagues. Whenever a student sat in on my clinic or attended my endoscopy list, I always asked: 'Any doctor relatives?' The answer was affirmative in at least half. It takes bottom to pick up a house officer or student for sloppiness when their parents were your classmates.

Mr Wolfe

The start of a three-day weekend on call – 'on take' – for general medicine. No such weekend passed without an email or phone call from medical manpower. It arrived at 10.00 a.m. on Friday. An intern rostered to be on call had 'mixed up' a swap, and there was no cover for the evening: 'I swapped my weekend nights,' he wrote, 'but accidentally swapped for a weekend I was already scheduled to work.' There was something puzzling, even post-modern, about this explanation. 'I tried my utmost,' he explained, 'to sort the issue, without any success.'

The endoscopy nurses asked me if I would carry out a gastroscopy on an inpatient. Sure. When the man was wheeled into the procedure room, I asked him what the problem was. 'Swallowing,' he said, pointing to his throat. I explained that I could not go ahead with the procedure, because people with this symptom should have a barium swallow X-ray first to make sure there wasn't a pharyngeal pouch. These pouches,* if unrecognised, are easily ruptured at endoscopy, with disastrous consequences, as I knew from personal experience. The man accepted my explanation without rancour, but his consultant flew into a rage.

'He hasn't got a pouch!' he screamed.

'How do you know?'

'Because I just *know*!'

Being 'on take' for general medicine over a long weekend reminded me of *Pulp Fiction*. A gangster is accidentally shot by two other hoodlums, Vincent (John Travolta) and Jules (Samuel L. Jackson). They take the body to their friend Jimmie's house. Jimmie (Quentin Tarantino) is enraged, shouting unprintable abuse at them. Vincent and Jules's boss, Marsellus (Ving Rhames), sends Mr Wolfe (Harvey Keitel) to deal with it. He is curt but polite and businesslike: 'I'm Winston Wolfe. I solve problems. Now you've got a corpse in a car, minus a head, in a garage. Take me to it.' Swiftly, efficiently and unfussily, Wolfe directs the disposal of the body and the removal of all traces of the event from the car.

---

* The pharynx is that part of the throat between the mouth and the oesophagus. Judge Jeffreys, the 'hanging judge' who presided over the 'Bloody Assizes' in the wake of Monmouth's rebellion in 1685, was said to have had a pharyngeal pouch. His bad temper and severe sentences were attributed to the constant regurgitation of decomposing food; Jeffreys had a spoon specially designed to extract food from the pouch.

Wolfe, according to the film producer Justin Szlasa, is a model of efficiency under pressure. He wrote an essay in 2012 entitled 'Being Winston Wolfe: 9 Reasons Why "Pulp Fiction" is the Management Guide Every Indie Filmmaker Needs'. Among the lessons Szlasa listed are: 1. Be 100% reliable; 2. Prioritise; 3. Bad news first; 4. Take things off your manager's plate – then own it; 5. Write things down; 6. Strategy is for amateurs, tactics are for professionals; 7. You can't manage what you don't understand; 8. Start tough, then soften up; 9. If it's not working, end it.

I'm tempted to do something similar for one of the medical journals: 'The conduct of the post-take round in general medicine: lessons from *Pulp Fiction*'s Mr Wolfe'.

General medicine was the dustbin of the ministry; a professional cul-de-sac, drained of interest, resource and prestige. This was the one clinical activity my colleagues immediately abandoned if the opportunity arose for them to do so. To address the trolley crisis, the ministry had opened two new units, the medical short-stay unit (MSSU) and the acute medical assessment unit (AMAU). These wards were staffed by a group of young physicians who specialised in 'acute medicine'. The MSSU, as its name suggests, took patients whose hospital stay was predicted to be short, while the AMAU was a curious hybrid of outpatient clinic and ward, where the GPs could send patients they were particularly worried about for 'rapid assessment'. Some patients sent to the AMAU were admitted, but most were sent home. These initiatives did not alleviate the trolley problem; the acute physicians cherry-picked those patients likely to be 'turned around' and discharged quickly, leaving all the other patients – the majority – with messier, less easily soluble problems to 'general medicine'. The MSSU did, however, produce data – demonstrating its short 'average length of stay' – that appealed to the managers and the politicians.

I took all the patients the specialists didn't want (which was most of them), those whose problems couldn't be neatly boxed, the old people who lacked rehabilitation potential. The 'easy' patients, who could be quickly 'processed' and discharged, were given beds in the MSSU, while the sick ones were left on trolleys in the emergency department, a cruel irony of the new iron managerialism, which viewed the metric of 'average length of stay' as more important than the care of the sick.

The worst thing about being a doctor is other doctors. The intense pressure led to squabbling; resentment piled on resentment. Academic disputes are famously bitter because there is so little at stake; medical disputes are bitter because there is so *much* at stake. Over a weekend on general medical 'take', there were multiple provocations to react like *Pulp Fiction*'s Jimmie, which I occasionally did, to my shame and regret. For many doctors at the ministry, it seemed that the most important question when confronted in the emergency department with a new sick patient was not what is wrong with this patient, or what immediate treatment would be best, but instead, *how can I move this patient on to another doctor?* The wise path, the skilful path, was Mr Wolfe's; unflappability is the greatest attribute a doctor can have. William Osler* called this 'imperturbability' or *aequanimitas*: 'Imperturbability means coolness and presence of mind under all circumstances, calmness amid storm, clearness of judgment in moments of grave peril, immobility, impassiveness, or, to use an old and expressive word, *phlegm*. It is the quality which is most appreciated by the laity though often misunderstood by them; and the physician who has the misfortune to be without it, who betrays indecision and worry, and who shows that he is flustered and flurried in ordinary emergencies, rapidly loses the confidence of his patients.' Osler, although he conceded that dealing with other physicians was 'often a testy and choleric business', was a fervent advocate for 'fellowship', or collegiality, among doctors. He liked to quote his hero, Sir Thomas Browne (author of *Religio Medici*): 'When thou lookest upon the imperfections of others, allow one eye for what is laudable in them.' I confess I could not consistently follow Osler's exhortations on 'fellowship'; I wonder if a long post-take round at the ministry would have breached his famous 'imperturbability'?

---

* Sir William Osler (1849–1919) was a Canadian physician, educator and writer. He was professor of medicine successively at McGill University, Montreal (1874–84), the University of Pennsylvania (1884–9), Johns Hopkins Hospital, Baltimore (1889–1905), and Oxford University (1905–19). He was an inspirational teacher, who established the first residency programme for the training of junior doctors and pioneered 'bedside' teaching of medical students. He introduced both grand rounds and journal clubs. His *Principles and Practice of Medicine* (1892) remains the most influential medical textbook ever written. He is often called – with some justification – 'The Father of Modern Medicine'.

Osler almost single-handedly established the model for how medicine is still practised and taught, yet his instincts were as much literary as scientific: he was a *humanist*, in the scholarly sense of that word. He did not, unfortunately, wear his learning lightly. His biographer Michael Bliss wrote: 'His style became more self-consciously literary, not always to good effect. He indulged his lifelong penchant for quotation, simile, and metaphor, burdening some of his reflections to the point where meaning becomes obscure and readers and listeners run away perplexed.'

Freud, a contemporary of Osler's, was, at heart, a literary man too. Eric Strauss and Richard Asher were typical of the next generation of medical humanists. But medicine no longer has a place for people like Osler, Freud, Strauss and Asher; would Nicky Haslam* regard it as a very *common* career?

Sitting in my office at 6.00 p.m. on a Friday evening, I wondered how many nights and weekends I had done over thirty-six years. I thought of a teacher friend, who had never worked a weekend or a bank holiday, who spent three months every summer by the sea with his children, and who radiated the serenity of the Buddha.

⌣

* Nicky Haslam – interior decorator and 'socialite' – used to write a newspaper column called 'How common'; the list of unpardonable vulgarities included 'loving your parents' (you love *nanny*) and 'being Scottish'.

On my way home, I walked through the hospital grounds; I found a small enclosed padlocked garden, neat and manicured, with a little gravel path. A sign proclaimed it 'James's Garden'. Who was James? I surmised that he was young, that he had died at the hospital, that he was much loved.

'I provide strictly spiritual services'

The 'post-take' round began in the emergency department at 7.00 a.m. The usual chaos and squalor; it took three hours to see all the new patients. Like Mr Wolfe, I liked to get the bad news first: 'How many do we have to see? Anyone in resus?'

Many of my patients had been admitted by the 'day' team, who had now finished their shift and gone home; last night's team, who did the early morning round with me, did not know them, so I had to carry out a full history and physical examination on each of these patients, a laborious exercise. (Incidentally, at weekends, the junior doctors on call with me were rarely members of my regular 'team'.)

A senior house officer began presenting one such patient by hesitantly reading from the notes.

'Have you seen this patient?' I asked.

'No. She was admitted by the day team.'

'So you don't know her?'

'No.'

*

A young Frenchwoman, on holiday in Ireland, was admitted to the clinical decision unit of the emergency department – supposedly a rapid-transit ward for minor complaints – with a severe kidney infection. She was now acutely unwell, shaking (rigoring) with fever, her blood pressure dropping. She had been given oral antibiotics, but clearly needed intra-venous treatment. She and her boyfriend were shocked by the field hospital environment and ask me if they could just fly back to Paris. I persuaded her to stay. I phoned my friend Con, the consultant on call for microbiology, to ask him for advice on the most suitable antibiotic. I apologised for calling so early: 'I'm phoning you from the seventh circle of hell.'

A man sent in from a nursing home with a worsening of his emphysema was now in respiratory failure. The registrar asked me if we should consider 'escalation' of his care – by which she meant admission to the intensive care unit – if he got worse. Unusually, his notes contained an advance directive, which made it quite clear that he wished for comfort measures only. 'Sorry, I didn't see that,' the registrar said.

The senior house officer presented the case of an elderly man and concluded that he had a 'lower respiratory tract infection'. This was unlikely because his chest X-ray was clear. The diagnosis of the admitting doctor had a strange potency; the narrative of 'the *pneumonia* in cubicle 7' almost unalterable, even when it became clear that that patient did *not* have pneumonia. This type of cognitive error is called 'diagnosis momentum': once a diagnostic label has been assigned to a patient by another individual, it is difficult to remove that label. Sick people were often referred to like this in the ministry: 'the pneumonia in cubicle 7'.

A ninety-year-old man, a childless widower, had been seen yesterday in the emergency department by the frailty intervention therapy team (FITT). They decided that he did not require admission, that he could go home 'with enhanced community support'. FITT was a new service set up by the geriatricians. Frail old people who turned up at the emergency department were assessed successively by the geriatrics registrar, a physiotherapist and an occupational therapist, with the idea of getting them out of the emergency department, out of the hospital and home, with the fabled 'enhanced community support'. Mission statement: 'The FITT aims for early therapy, identification, assessment and intervention of frail adults over 75 years to facilitate safe and early discharge from the ED [emergency department] setting.'

The FITT therapists wrote comprehensive accounts of this man's domestic circumstances and medical issues. A few hours after this assessment, his niece brought him back to the emergency department, where he became *my* responsibility; he would *not* be admitted under geriatrics: they had washed their hands of him. Although his mobility had gradually deteriorated over the past several weeks, there was no *acute* illness, and he did not need urgent hospitalisation. The 'problem' was a disagreement between the old man and his niece as to whether he should continue living alone at home or go to a nursing home. The best way of resolving this impasse, she decided, was to abandon the old man in the emergency department.

When we finally finished, we were tired, hungry and thirsty, but the canteen was closed. I met a hospital chaplain on the corridor outside the canteen, and jokingly asked if he wouldn't mind brewing a pot of tea. 'I provide strictly spiritual services,' he replied gravely.

The chaplain and I had been to the same school; he was a few years older than me but looked younger, having kept both his hair and his boyish enthusiasm. He had been a star player in the team that won the national schools' hurling championship in 1974. His trajectory from hurler to priest was what the seminary school prided itself in, academic attainment being of lesser importance.

At 12.30, I joined the telephone conference convened by the clinical director. I listened to tedious accounts of the number of patients presenting to the emergency department who required admission (too many), the number of patients discharged (too few), the bed status in the satellite rural hospitals, whether any CT or MRI scans were required, how many intensive care unit beds were available. A woman representing one of the satellite rural hospitals had a piercing, unpleasant voice, so loud I had to hold the phone some distance from my ear. I drifted off during this litany of woe, only to be woken by the clinical director:

'Seamus, are there any patients from last night suitable for transfer?' (By this he meant transfer to one of the satellite hospitals.) One old lady admitted under my care lived near one of these hospitals, and *might* have been suitable, but I couldn't summon the energy to track down whomever was on call there for medicine, to go back to the woman and see if she was willing, and then phone the bed offices in both hospitals.

'No, no one suitable,' I lied.

A stranger in a strange land

Another heavy 'take'. Most of my patients were accommodated upstairs on the floor over the emergency department in the AMAU (acute medical assessment unit), a five-day unit designed for outpatients, not as a general medical *ward*. When the weekend take became even more unmanageable than usual, the bed managers opened the AMAU, and general medical patients were 'decanted'* into it. This was mainly driven by centrally imposed targets: the ministry was fined if any patient over seventy-five was on a trolley for more than seven hours in the emergency department.

The AMAU doctors and nurses got very annoyed if they came in on a Monday morning and found their unit full of elderly frail general medical patients – cuckoos, as they saw it, in their nest. There was this sense throughout the ministry that patients must be somehow *deserving* of the ward they were sent to, that a patient, say, with pneumonia, sent to the stroke ward was an unworthy interloper, that they shouldn't

* A word as dehumanising as 'the pneumonia in cubicle 7'.

be admitted to this exclusive club. This contempt extended to their doctors too: what was this *gastroenterologist* doing on our cystic fibrosis ward?

When I and the team of three junior doctors arrived in the AMAU at 7.00 a.m., the night nurses sent there from the emergency department were still on duty. Several were lounging at the nurses' station, one in a full Jacob Rees-Mogg reclining pose.

'Would any of you like to go around with us?' I asked.

'If you want,' said Rees-Mogg grudgingly.

My first patient was a Lithuanian woman of forty, who had recently been diagnosed with lung cancer. She had been through the respiratory and oncology services and was now consigned to general medicine. The entire right side of her body was paralysed: this was caused by secondary cancer deposits in her brain. She had no husband, partner or relatives, and spoke little English. A kindly neighbour held her hand. She would die soon, a stranger in a strange land, without family or friends, moved along like a parcel from one medical service to the next. I was examining her lifeless limbs when a nurse opened the curtain. 'Bed management says you're to transfer at least three.'

'I'm kind of busy.'

'I'm only passing on a message.'

A querulous eighty-five-year-old woman, in respiratory failure from emphysema and pneumonia, and wearing a tight-fitting mask that forced oxygen into her cigarette-ravaged lungs. She couldn't – she wouldn't – wear the mask, she said, it was too uncomfortable.

'She keeps pulling it off,' said Rees-Mogg, 'and her oxygen saturations drop.'

'Let her be,' I said. I thought – but did not say – she'll die anyway; why worry about her oxygen saturations?

A man of only fifty-five with advanced dementia, admitted now with seizures. Although 'new onset of epilepsy' was an indisputable 'category A' admission* to neurology, the consultant neurologist on call had refused to take him, arguing that the man's dementia made him a general medical patient.

The young French tourist was still sick; too sick to protest, too sick to entertain thoughts of escaping to Paris.

A man with chest pain. Although he had known heart disease, the cardiology registrar refused to take him until we (the doctors on call for general medicine) had 'out-ruled a pulmonary embolus' (lung clot). Junior doctors attached to specialist services became obsessed with their gatekeeper role; did they get a dressing-down from their consultants if an unworthy 'general' patient slipped through on their watch? Or was it just laziness and disobligingness? I phoned the consultant cardiologist on call, who agreed to take the patient.

---

* Meaning a diagnosis or presenting symptom that (supposedly) mandated admission under that speciality.

*

Another super-tanker patient belonging to my saintly colleague. This woman spent at least half the year in the hospital
and attended the outpatients every week. I waded through the
multi-volume case notes; her diagnosis was a label conferred
on her after a visit to London to see a private consultant who
specialised in this rare, and, to some, dubious, disease. She
was admitted now with a minor chest infection, which could
have been treated at home, but her GP, fearful of both the
super-tanker and the rare disease, sent her in. She had been
started – appropriately – on an oral antibiotic but wasn't happy
with this treatment.

'I normally get Taz when I've got a chest infection,' she
said, deploying the slangy 'Taz' – for the intravenous antibiotic
Tazocin – to make it quite clear that she knew all about these
things, that she was not to be fobbed off, like some civilian,
with *tablets*. I looked at her clear chest X-ray and normal blood
tests. 'Sure. No problem.'

'The team are an absolute disgrace'

Monday: my third consecutive post-take round, and another 7.00 a.m. start. On my way to the emergency department, I met a cleaner who told me that there had been a flood in the basement, the generator was down, the lights were out in the intensive care unit, there were fire engines at the back door. Too good to be true, I thought.

I now had fifty-two patients. My first was an alcoholic Russian admitted with withdrawal seizures and pneumonia. Heavily sedated, he barely noticed my presence. The case notes told the usual story of broken bones and *delirium tremens*; I read the many earnest and optimistic assessments by the alcohol liaison nurses.

There was a daily meeting on weekdays at 8.30 a.m. to discuss the previous night's 'take'. I rarely attended; I usually sent my registrar. This gathering, chaired by one of the MSSU acute physicians, was meant to move some of the new admissions on to other departments; geriatrics, for example, *might* take two patients, provided they were not *too sick*. Although it lasted for only ten or fifteen minutes, I couldn't bear the thought of this Potemkin exercise; sitting in an airless room with the bed managers and representatives from the other medical units so that two or three of my patients could be moved on. Occasionally – when I had a sick patient with a problem beyond my expertise – this made sense, but these were generally the very patients the other departments declined to take over. Mr Wolfe (the clean-up guy) would have had nothing to do with this.

By 9.30 a.m., I had walked (according to my smartphone) 9,863 steps; my patients were scattered across fifteen wards and corridors. As I walked out of the front door on the way to my office, I passed a man talking loudly on his phone: 'The team are an absolute disgrace,' he said. When I arrived at my office, I shut my eyes for five minutes, then opened the emails. A message from my secretary: a relative of one of the inpatients had phoned demanding an 'urgent meeting with the team before 2 p.m.'. Somehow, I *knew* that this relative was the man I had passed at the front door a few minutes before. The only way to defuse this situation would be for me to see him, rather than delegating this task to my registrar. This meant that I would miss the X-ray conference, particularly important today, after a weekend on 'take', when so many scans and X-rays had to be reviewed.

It *was* the man at the front door. I explained to him that it wasn't always possible for me to see relatives, particularly on a day like this, when I had to see so many patients, attend an X-ray conference, and then do an endoscopy list. I usually saw relatives, I told him, at designated times during ward rounds. 'But nobody told me that,' he said sweetly.

He questioned me in some detail about his elderly father's many problems. I spent thirty minutes with him when I should have been reviewing the X-rays and scans of my many other patients. He was cunning. He did not raise his voice – in fact, he smiled throughout.* He probed with the subtlety of a barrister. What was his father's potassium level? Why had he been changed from intravenous to oral antibiotics? Did his chest X-ray show any sign of pulmonary oedema? When the cross-examination finally concluded, he expressed a conditional, grudging satisfaction.

I went to the endoscopy unit and switched off my phone. I thought about this encounter. Would I be more attentive to the father now because of the attentions of his son? Were my many other patients any concern of his? I felt like the maître d' of a bad restaurant sent out to apologise for the lousy food and sloppy service.

⌒

The endoscopy nurses told me that a legless man – a double amputee – had come in three days before for a colonoscopy. He informed them that there was no one to collect him after the procedure, and he wasn't willing to have it without sedation. Patients who had been sedated had to be picked up

---

* Medical secretaries often told me that relatives and patients would scream and swear at them, but when they met the *doctors* face to face, they were meek and polite.

and accompanied home by 'a responsible person'. They told him they couldn't go ahead and sent him home in a taxi. When he got home, his daughter wouldn't let him in. The taxi driver brought him back to the hospital, where he spent the weekend on a trolley in the emergency department.

I passed a man on the footpath to my office who had once been my patient. He was one of the few people I had ever encountered who was *evil*, whose mere presence sucked out my spirit. He had retired from his undemanding job some years before on the grounds of chronic fatigue. He looked well as he walked briskly past. I was relieved he did not recognise me.

An email from a friend, asking if I wanted to attend a lecture in Edinburgh by the doctor-novelist Abraham Verghese; his talk would be on 'the physician as revolutionary'. I cannot think of a profession *less* revolutionary than medicine.

'They usually put them under general medicine when they die in resus'

A man in his thirties, at the smokers' corner near the main entrance, was on his phone, shouting, smoking. His face was crimson with fresh abrasions. Apart from a blanket draped over his shoulders, his only clothing was tracksuit bottoms. He was shoeless.

The Tuesday after a weekend on 'take' was often the busiest day; I had to see all the patients admitted over the weekend *and* all the patients I already had before the weekend. My list was now down to forty-two patients in fifteen locations.

We spoke of 'the ministry' as if it had a personality: the ministry did this, but neglected that, people said, as if it was an unpredictable, capricious parent. I often complained that the ministry made my work difficult by allocating so many patients to my care, and then scattering them over multiple, often highly unsuitable, locations. If one were to design a system to maximise error and poor communication, I would say, you could not do better. The banal truth was that there was no such personality, neither capricious nor consistent; there was no great designer. The ministry was a market where the major commodity being traded was responsibility; I was currently overinvested in this negative currency.

You *had* to do a ward round in the morning: if you got around early, it gave the team time to do their individual tasks – the 'jobs' – and, because visiting hours were in the afternoon, you were not slowed down by relatives wanting to talk. Theteamareanabsolutedisgrace, however, was not one to be daunted by official visiting times and was by his father's bedside when I arrived. I checked his progress with the team; the old man was slowly improving. As I was walking away, the son came after me.

'Aren't you going to examine his chest to check for fluid overload?'

'Of course,' I said, and went back to sound out the old man's chest with my stethoscope.

The man discharged by the FITT team was now, ironically, in the geriatric ward, but still under my care. His 'old' case notes, which were 'missing' over the weekend, were now available. He had attended the geriatric clinic on numerous occasions; his case notes were full of long, worthy, solicitous letters from this service to his GP. One letter listed poly-pharmacy* as number eight in a list of twelve 'problems', itemising the sixteen medications he was taking. Mindful though they were of their long-standing concern for his welfare, the geriatricians would take him on now, they said, only if he displayed 'rehabilitation potential'. They concluded regretfully that he was distinctly lacking in this quality.

My registrar told me that the mortuary had phoned, asking one of the team to sign a death certificate.

'But we had no deaths over the weekend,' I said.

'Actually, we *did*. A woman came into the emergency department on Friday night with a huge brain haemorrhage. She died within an hour of coming in.'

'I never heard anything about her.'

'They usually put them under general medicine when they die in resus.'

A woman, not my patient, who had been on the ward for many weeks, sat at the nurses' station. Demented patients were sometimes placed there; for some reason, it often calmed them. This woman sat there, sometimes for several hours, tapping the desk with her hand, saying 'downtown, downtown,' over and over, in her low, almost masculine, smoker's voice. Every time I visited the ward, I heard 'downtown, downtown'. Where all the lights are bright.

* The consumption of five or more medications every day.

I went through the case notes of a man who had been an inpatient six months before, and was now suing the hospital – and me, presumably. Although he had been under my care for less than twenty-four hours, I had seen him soon after admission and carefully documented my findings and my plan for him. The alleged failure was to do with a scan, and beyond my control. I read the notes with intense relief.

The Irish are by nature litigious. When I came back to the ministry in 2001, a colleague warned me: 'You must keep in mind that although we have *Albanian* infrastructure, we have *American* litigation.'

I watched my elderly sick cat being euthanised. The vet did it so gently, so humanely, with such *kindness*, that it made me reconsider my opposition to it in humans. I wondered if this resistance was genuine, or was it driven by my visceral dislike of its proponents, and their odious, hectoring certainty?

'There's a lot of it about'

I crept in via the back door of the lecture theatre for the grand round. Despite several prominent signs stating that 'no food or drink is to be consumed in the lecture theatre', most of the audience were bovinely munching on sandwiches and slurping on coffee handed out by a drug rep who had set up a food stand by the main entrance. No grand round, it seemed, could proceed without such industry-sponsored victuals. An exception was a lecture on death I had given a few years before. A colleague, lamenting the absence of food, observed that *death* was clearly something the pharmaceutical industry was not keen to promote.

The speaker was a newly appointed orthogeriatrician, who specialised in the rehabilitation of elderly people who had broken their hips. His slides showed an 'exponential rise' in the number of old people cracking their hips. *Everything* was rising exponentially: autism, depression, Crohn's disease, osteoporosis, cancer. The world would soon be a vast clinic, populated only by patients and health workers. The presentation concluded that the solution to this epidemic of broken hips was investment in orthogeriatric services.

On my way to clinic, I spotted the ministry's most notorious super-tanker patient. Hunched, he clung to a drip stand, smoking and talking loudly on his phone. Malice exuded from every atom of his tiny frame. He had spent most of the last five years in the hospital with a condition – or, rather, a 'constellation of symptoms' – that no one could bring together in a unifying diagnosis. He talked and bullied his many doctors into a multitude of tests and treatments, including several operations. His case, documented in several large volumes of notes, was now so complex that no single doctor could be entirely sure what had been done to him. There had been multiple meetings with a variety of agencies, and several attempts to discharge him, but they had all failed, usually at the eleventh hour. Any hope of cure, or even amelioration, had been abandoned. Now, the emphasis was on containment, on fencing off this intractable problem, on sharing around the pain and the responsibility. I had a sneaking admiration for his ability to manipulate every professional with whom he came in contact. Resourceful and cunning, he was stronger than the ministry. I counted it as one of the triumphs of my career that I had never dealt with him.

The first outpatient was a demented woman with 'halitosis'. Her GP wanted me to 'exclude helicobacter* infection'. The poor woman's bad breath was due to her rotten teeth and gums. Her daughter was unimpressed with this diagnosis, however, and insisted that I do a breath test for *Helicobacter*. I booked it, knowing that she might not be able to do this test, which, like a breathalyser test for drink-driving, required some degree of comprehension and co-ordination.

A woman of fifty-five, dressed like a teenager in a pink track-suit and trainers, and busy on her laptop when I called her in.

'I've been diagnosed with Ehlers-Danlos† syndrome,' she said.

'Oh,' I replied with that non-judgemental, non-committal tone I had honed over many years.

'What do you think about Ehlers-Danlos syndrome?' she asked.

I paused. This once rare condition was now being diagnosed with alarming frequency, on the flimsiest of criteria, mainly by consultants working in full-time private practice.

'There's a lot of it about.'

*

---

* *Helicobacter pylori* is a bacterium usually found in the stomach; it infects more than half the world's population. Although it is associated with gastritis, ulcers (gastric and duodenal) and stomach cancer, it is harmless in most people infected with it.

† Ehlers-Danlos syndrome (or *syndromes*) are a group of rare inherited conditions that affect the skin and joints, and (occasionally) the gut.

A woman gave me a pamphlet from a colonic irrigation* 'clinic'. The 'clinic' was housed in the front room of a suburban semi-detached house, but then, so were most GP surgeries in the vicinity of the ministry. This brochure was entitled 'Death begins in the colon: toxins produced in the bowels and re-absorbed into the body can devastate your health'. Colonic irrigation, it said, 'is a pleasant and relaxing experience'. The patient's 'irrigationist' had told her that she had *Helicobacter pylori* infection; she could diagnose this, she said, by the colour of the *effluent* – it was always *green*.

* Colonic irrigation seems to have declined as a fad since its heyday in the 1990s; I wonder if this was related to the demise of its most famous devotee, Princess Diana. It also attracted bad publicity when a few unfortunate 'patients' had their colons perforated by the tube used to irrigate them and had to undergo emergency surgery.

Colonic irrigation has had something of a comeback recently on the back of all the modish 'microbiome' research (the role of gut bacteria in human disease).

'... it is high time that Mr Bunbury made up his mind whether he was going to live or die'

World Sepsis Day: 'a global health crisis'.

Theteamareanabsolutedisgrace was waiting for me on the ward round. We played a cagey game, but he eventually caught me out when he asked about his father's brain CT. I did not know that the patient had been for this scan; after a quick, nervous conference with my registrar, I reassured the son that apart from a little age-related atrophy, it was clear. The patient asked if he could go home. Theteamareanabsolutedisgrace held his father's hand, and in his creepy, simpering voice, said: 'I'm not sure about that, Dad.'

'You go home when you *both* feel ready,' I said, grabbing the opportunity to escape.

*

I next saw Mr Jones, the man who had been admitted two months before with a fractured pelvis, and who was now – very slowly – dying. He had been 'lodging' in the cardiac renal building since admission; the word 'lodging' implied that he did not *deserve* to be in this beautiful new building, because he had an illness that was neither cardiac nor renal. He was still alive, still *not dead*, two weeks after being declared to be – in the oxymoronic phrase – 'actively dying'. Like Bunbury in *The Importance of Being Earnest*, 'the doctors found out that he could not live'. He was now in a single room, semi-conscious, his breathing laboured and irregular. His family members patiently maintained their vigil. There was nothing to say; we were all vaguely embarrassed that he was still alive. Like Charles II, he was taking 'a most unconscionable time a-dying'. The palliative care doctors had started him on a syringe driver, delivering morphine and sedation, but Mr Jones clung on. Families commonly believed that the syringe driver *killed* people; not so, said the palliative care doctors – it merely made dying more 'comfortable'. I wondered; the commencement of the syringe driver nearly always signalled the imminence of death. But still he did not oblige. Unlike Bunbury, Mr Jones did not seem to have great confidence in the opinions of his physicians.

It was catching, this not-dying, this defiance of the doctors' prognostications. On the last round, I had confidently informed the daughter of a ninety-five-year-old woman – who came in with pneumonia – that I did not expect her to survive. Now I was telling her we were planning to send her back to her nursing home.

*

I suggested to a man in his late sixties, who had completed ten days' antibiotic treatment for a chest infection, that he might go home. He and his wife looked alarmed, mentioning several new symptoms, including neck pain and dizziness. They were also worried, they told me, about his high blood sugar. This was almost certainly caused by steroids, which he had taken for five years; neither he nor I knew why he was on this medication. I excused myself and sat down at the desk with his notes. The steroids had been started years before, when he was acutely ill with pneumonia; they should have been stopped when he went home, but no one thought to do this. His GP dutifully renewed the prescription every few months. Five years on, the steroids, as well as making him diabetic, had ravaged his bones and skin, and made him easy prey to infection.

The man's case notes documented his numerous admissions under various services; since 2008, he had undergone 900 blood tests and seventy X-rays and scans. Although he had blockages in the arteries of his legs, emphysema, and a mini stroke (following which he had an operation to unblock his carotid artery), he continued to smoke. Perhaps he *needed* to keep smoking: being sick was his full-time occupation; health would have been ruinous.

~

The ministry's 'sepsis champion', an anaesthetist, was manning a stand in the canteen, raising awareness of sepsis, a campaign to which the entire week had been dedicated. His presence reminded me that the word 'septic' in Cork slang means 'conceited'. We nodded curtly; he was aware of my views on the sepsis mania, with its unbeatable combination of bad medicine and aggressive marketing.* I had coffee with

---

* 'Sepsis', which used to be called 'infection', can mean many things, from a pneumonia in an elderly patient to life-threatening blood poisoning (septicaemia) in a child. The former scenario is far more common: most deaths attributed to 'sepsis' occur in frail old people. Sepsis awareness campaigns began because of some rare cases of preventable deaths in children and young adults, such as that of Rory Staunton, a twelve-year-old boy from New York who died in 2012 after a minor cut (sustained at basketball) became infected and led to septicaemia. These campaigns stressed the importance of early administration of antibiotics and a low threshold for the diagnosis. This led to the formulation of very flimsy tickbox criteria for the diagnosis of sepsis, which resulted in many people being treated for sepsis who did not have it. Many doctors are openly critical of this awareness campaign, the new diagnostic criteria and the mandatory sepsis treatment protocols. Professor Mervyn Singer and colleagues from the Bloomsbury Institute of Intensive Care Medicine at University College Hospital, London, wrote to *The Lancet* on 26 October 2019:

'"Sepsis kills over 52,000 every year – each death a preventable tragedy", tweeted Matt Hancock, UK Secretary of State for Health and Social Care, in March 2019. Many other non-contextualised or fictitious claims regularly fill media pages and airwaves, creating a distorted picture of sepsis epidemiology and unrealistic expectation of outcomes. This hype has generated an unhealthy climate of fear and retribution in both the UK and the USA.

'... the high incidence of frailty and severe comorbidities makes most sepsis-related deaths neither attributable to sepsis, nor preventable through timely and effective health care.

'... The Surviving Sepsis Campaign strongly recommends antimicrobial [antibiotic] administration within an hour of presentation, contending that each hour's delay costs lives. However, the evidence base is underwhelming and openly challenged by the Infectious Diseases Society of America, among others.

'... A spike in sepsis-coded deaths coincided with the implementation in April 2017, of new NHS Digital Coding Guidance and with financial incentives to code a patient's diagnosis as sepsis. A similar effect has been noted in the USA. Furthermore, up to 40% of patients initially diagnosed as having sepsis were later judged as not likely to be infected.'

a microbiologist, who told me that since this sepsis campaign began, the number of blood cultures (to detect infection in the bloodstream, so-called septicaemia) sent to his laboratory had doubled; the number of 'positive' blood cultures, however, did not alter. He shared my views on the sepsis campaign but thought resistance was futile.

An email announcing the sixth National Sepsis Summit; this year's theme is: 'Could it be sepsis?' A strange question, rhetorical rather than Socratic. There were two possible answers: first, yes, 'it' *could* be sepsis (although it probably *isn't*); second, no, 'it' could be a hundred other things.

The sepsis bandwagon, however, seemed to be immune to these well-argued criticisms, and retained the unqualified support of the politicians, the hospital managers, the World Health Organization and the ministry's 'sepsis champion'.

'The valves of Haustra?'

On call again, the fourth in seven nights. Not a big 'take', but all the new patients were *sick*, and all were on trolleys arranged in a line; this trail of tears now stretched as far as the café adjoining the emergency department. The presence of trolleys near or even *within* the café was an unofficial (but widely accepted) metric for a special level of awfulness within the emergency department.

Daithi, a man in his fifties, with a history of cancer – for which he had a lung removed two years before – came in with the highest blood calcium I had ever seen. He was at high risk of cardiac arrest; we needed to lower his calcium levels quickly with intravenous fluids and a drug called Zometa.

After the round, I went on to my endoscopy list but was phoned, as I was doing the first procedure, by an emergency department nurse, complaining that she couldn't contact *any* member of my team, and that Daithi was much worse. I felt obliged both to take the call and to apologise to my current patient for taking it. I phoned my registrar and told him to attend to Daithi immediately. He mentioned in passing that Mr Jones (Bunbury) had finally died. What should he put down in the death certificate? I told him it would be better if he did *not* write 'fractured pelvis' as the *primary* cause of death, lest this attract the attentions of the coroner. Yes, of course he should put it down, I said, but only as a *contributory* factor.

A medical student attended my list: 'observing a colonoscopy' was a requirement for the final year, a box to be ticked. I pointed to the mucosal folds in the rectum and asked what they were called. He didn't know.

'Don't worry. I've asked that question of every medical student who came to watch a colonoscopy, and in twenty years, not one has known the answer. They're called the valves of Houston.'*

He stayed for the next colonoscopy.

'So what are those folds in the rectum called?'

'The valves of Haustra?'

I called into the hospice on the way home to see a relative.

* John Houston (1802–45) was an Irish surgeon and anatomist. He was also interested in zoology and wrote a paper 'On the structure and mechanism of the tongue of the chameleon'.

As I walked in the main entrance, a nurse passed, pushing a wheelchair in which sat a smiling elderly man. He was the professor of psychiatry when I was an undergraduate. One of his teaching methods was to film one of the students interviewing a patient. I gamely volunteered. My patient was a taciturn elderly man with depression, then known as 'involutional melancholia'.

'I've done terrible things,' he said.

'What things?' I asked.

He shook his head: 'No, I couldn't tell you. I wouldn't want people to know.'

'Don't worry, *nobody* will hear. Whatever you tell me is *completely confidential*. There's only the two of us here,' I reassured him, as my classmates erupted with laughter in the adjoining room.

When I returned to the tutorial room, the professor sat there for some time, with the same beatific smile, and eventually turned to me and said: 'Zero marks for interview technique.'

I came in the next morning – a Saturday – even though I was not on call; I was worried about Daithi: that no one would routinely check on him, that when I came in on Monday morning, someone would tell me that he had died. Sick patients were not routinely reviewed over the weekend by the physician on call, who saw only the *new* admissions. For that reason, I often had to come in at weekends when not on call; this was a burden to which I had never entirely reconciled myself. Every Friday I would go around the wards, wondering if any patient was too sick to be left unseen for two days; there was nearly always at least one.

It was a glorious sunny autumn day; I hadn't had a day off in three weeks. Daithi was stable; his calcium was falling. I wrote a note in his chart, thinking how odd it was to be ever mindful that the note you wrote now, on your day off, might in a few years be forensically dissected by an expert hired by a litigating solicitor. To practise medicine is to have a permanent feeling that you've forgotten something.

'These things happen'

The first patient at the clinic had recently been to the neurology outpatients, where he had been given a label of 'chronic subjective dizziness'. I had never heard of this syndrome; presumably, it was thought to be more acceptable than 'unexplained dizziness', or 'idiopathic dizziness', or – worst of all – '*functional* dizziness', 'functional'* being a euphemism for symptoms without a physical cause. Some progressives have called for that use of the word to be banned.

Next, a man sent by a GP who referred rarely, but when he did, the patients were always 'challenging'. The man walked in, loudly burping.

'I don't have to tell you *my* problem!'

'How long has that been bothering you?' I asked hopefully.

* A gastroenterologist I trained with had a large private practice. When explaining to his fee-paying irritable bowel syndrome patients the nature of their condition, he always began: 'There are disorders of *structure*, and there are disorders of *function*. Yours is a disorder of function.'

'Forty years.'

'Any worse?'

'No,' he burped, 'saving your presence.'

�⟩

I did my round in the afternoon; the list was down to thirty patients in fourteen locations. Daithí's CT scan, as expected, showed recurrence of cancer in his bones, liver, brain, skull and spine. His spinal cord was in imminent danger of compression. He asked me to tell him the result of the scan. As I spoke to him, an alarm siren – somewhere, where? – went off. Do you want me to come back later? No, tell me now. The communication skills experts (like Dr Jack) might have used our conversation as a training video on 'how *not* to do it': Daithí was on a trolley, a flimsy screen the only privacy afforded him; no nurse came on the round; no friend or relative was with him. This difficult conversation, however, could not be postponed or fudged. He wanted, he *needed* to know. So I told him, my voice competing with the siren.

I think he already knew. Although he insisted that nothing be withheld, I tried to spare him the very worst details – such as the fact that his *skull* was full of cancer deposits. Like many recipients of such news, he immediately focused on the question of how *quickly* he could 'start treatment'. I didn't have the heart to tell him that any 'treatment' would be palliative, that if it were *me*, I would go home and spend whatever time left to me with my family. Such honesty is now impossible; it is too often construed as 'taking hope away'. How I wished we could have talked, not as 'doctor' and 'patient', but as two *men*.

Instead, I put my hand on his shoulder, and told him I would talk with the radiation specialist and the oncologist and get back to him 'with a plan'.

The man discharged by the FITT team was in good spirits. We had something in common: he had worked in the Ford assembly plant for thirty years; my father had worked there too. We chatted amiably about the people we knew there, the old corny jokes about the Ford's workers stealing parts: 'If you pushed him, he'd start!' The discharge co-ordinator documented her numerous 'challenging' encounters with his niece. I wrote a short entry in the notes, stating that he had the capacity to make his own decisions.

The discharge co-ordinators saw the very worst of human beings: their greed, their cruelty, their anger, the bizarre transmutations of guilt. Astonishingly, they were not weary misanthropes; they were cheerful, patient, always prepared to give families another chance, always willing to put a benign interpretation on the worst behaviour. The most senior discharge co-ordinator had been the clinical nurse manager on a ward where a family subjected the staff to a six-month-long campaign of bullying and abuse, yet when it finally ended with the death of their mother, she bore them no ill will. A year later, when the most vindictive of this family killed himself, she might have been entitled to a moment of grim satisfaction, but she felt only sorrow. She had forgiven him:

'God love him,' she said. She might have quite justifiably blamed the ministry for failing to protect her and her nurses, but did not; perhaps, like me, she did not believe that the ministry had a personality, much less a soul. 'These things happen,' she said. 'It's over now.'

A safety huddle

Yet another night of general medical on call, my fifth in eleven days. The senior house officer handed me the list of new patients; as usual, most of the admissions went to general medicine. An icon was attached to the admission list for each speciality: a brain for neurology, a heart for cardiology, some red blood cells for haematology. The icon for geriatrics was Carl Fredricksen,* the grumpy old man in the film *Up*; the geriatricians were reported to be unhappy with this symbol.

An elderly man, a retired civil servant, had been admitted with delirium, possibly caused by a viral infection of the brain (encephalitis). Unusually, he was confabulating in the Irish language, even though he was not a native speaker.

*

* Described by Richard Corliss of *Time* magazine as being like 'a disgruntled bear that's been poked awake during hibernation'.

A Scottish woman of fifty with a new lung cancer had disease *everywhere*: lung, brain, bones, neck lymph nodes. Oblivious of her situation, she cracked jokes as I examined the huge tumour lumps in her neck. This indifference, even frivolousness, was not uncommon; did nature, or some benign force, take pity on us? The house officer who presented her case used the very technical neurological term dysdiadochokinesia* to describe this woman's incoordination, caused by the cancer deposits in her brain. I remarked that this was the first time anyone had used that term on a 'post-take' general medical ward round; the house officer beamed with pride.

I went to see Daithi. I had asked the radiation specialists to see him with a view to irradiating his spine to prevent spinal cord compression. A consultant saw him but would agree to proceed with this only if a spinal surgeon first pronounced it *safe* to do so. I phoned a spinal surgeon – a friend – who promised he would see the patient. An oncologist had also been to see him but would not start chemotherapy until we had taken a biopsy to *prove* that this was a recurrence of his cancer, even though there was nothing else it could be.

⌣‿⌐

---

* Dysdiadochokinesia refers to the inability to perform rapid, alternating movement, such as flipping one's hand from back to front. It is a sign of disease in the cerebellum, the part of the brain situated in the back of the head that controls co-ordination.

I read a letter from a haematology consultant, advising me that a blood sample taken for 'cross-matching' (checking the blood type before transfusion) from one of my patients had been mislabelled, an error, she wrote, that might have had 'catastrophic consequences'. I requested the notes and found that this mislabelling had occurred at 3.00 a.m. on Easter Monday in the emergency department. The patient was an elderly woman admitted after a fall; she was on a trolley in a corridor when this sample was taken by the sleep-deprived duty house officer. Five months later, this was now *my* responsibility.

The grand round was on 'patient safety', and as Pharisaical as I had feared. The sepsis champion reluctantly admitted that there had been no fall in mortality from sepsis at the ministry since the introduction of the mandatory sepsis protocol. (He did not mention that the number of blood cultures sent to microbiology had doubled in that time, as had antibiotic usage.) This was followed by a video address by the director general of the World Health Organization, Dr Tedros Adhanom Ghebreyesus, who told us that famous monuments around the world, including the Egyptian pyramids and the statue of Christ the Redeemer in Rio de Janeiro, were to be lit up in orange to raise awareness of sepsis.*

* This awareness had now reached feverish proportions. The diagnosis could be made by tick box, with vague criteria, including confusion, breathlessness and a fast heart rate, symptoms that have numerous causes besides sepsis. These flimsy diagnostic criteria led to many of my patients being treated for sepsis who were not septic. Meanwhile, we were regularly

Next, a medication safety pharmacist, whose first PowerPoint slide proclaimed: 'Culture eats strategy for breakfast!' The final speaker was the new hospital chief executive, flanked by the clinical directors, who announced that he would carry out unscheduled 'quality and safety walk rounds'. Would he, I wondered, do a 'walk round' at 3.00 a.m. on a bank holiday in the emergency department to check on the safe labelling of blood samples?

An email from a speech and language therapist:

> Dear all
>
> We have been talking on the ward about the benefit of coming together to co-ordinate the care of complex patients. This is called a safety huddle. We are proposing we have 2 meet ups a week on Tuesday and Thursday at 11.30. Everyone is welcome. The aim will be to highlight any risks and to enable joint decision making to maximise patient care and expedite flow.

The world *huddle* conjured an excruciating image of comradely embraces from my fellow healthcare workers.

---

admonished by pharmacists and antibiotic 'stewards' that we were over-using antibiotics, and, if we were not careful, we would create a world where antibiotics would be ineffective because of bacterial resistance.

A random act of kindness

I had been on call so often lately that I forgot to reset my alarm, and I was woken at 5.30 a.m.

The first patient on my ward round that day was a demented old man, sent in with anaemia. His family members were content when I told them I would not do invasive tests (gastroscopy and colonoscopy) for this condition. Now in his late eighties, he had been diagnosed with pancreatic cancer – almost invariably fatal – twenty years before. An excellent surgeon had performed a palliative bypass operation to decompress the stomach, leaving the cancer untouched and intact. He wrote to the GP: 'I don't have tissue [meaning a biopsy], but I am confident of the diagnosis.' The only possible explanations were an incorrect diagnosis or a miracle. Why not a miracle?

I admired this surgeon: he had *bottom*. He always did the right thing: not the safe thing, or the thing demanded by protocols, or the convenient thing, but the *right* thing. He was the *anti*-free-rider: he embraced – even actively sought out – the difficult stuff. He once rebuked me for sending a patient with a complex bile duct problem to a Dublin hospital; I had assumed that this man would have to go to a unit that specialised in such problems. The surgeon told me that when he was a senior registrar in Glasgow, he had written up a large series of patients with this problem, and that he would have been happy to operate. Predictably, the specialist unit in Dublin cancelled the patient's surgery *twice*; he went back to his native country for the operation. 'Aren't you an awful eejit?' the surgeon said to me.

Daithi was the object of a game of pass-the-parcel played now by four services: mine, spinal surgery, radiotherapy and oncology. He was sent for a 'mapping' CT of his spine – to plan the radiation treatment – but had been inexplicably sent back from the X-ray department without this being done. He was confused, angry and frightened; who could blame him? My role was now that of messenger boy. I phoned the radiotherapy consultant, who said he *might* consider taking him over, but only after he had discussed this further with the oncologist and the spinal surgeon. 'Why don't the three of you have a chat among yourselves?' I suggested.

The Scottish woman with lung cancer had swapped the corridor of the emergency department for the corridor of the geriatric ward. The radiologists had taken a biopsy sample from her neck nodes. Her jauntiness had now evaporated. She asked me what was wrong with her. I wanted to tell her – she had a right to know; but as I looked at her, perched on a trolley in the loud, unforgiving ward corridor, I lost my nerve.

'We'll have to wait for that biopsy result.'

A woman who had been admitted with a chest infection was now jaundiced. I learned from her notes – unavailable at the time of admission – that she had had a similar episode of jaundice in 2016, attributed to an antibiotic, the same anti-biotic she was now on.

'We didn't have the notes when she came in,' my registrar pleaded in mitigation.

'But you had them yesterday.'

The man whose delirium expressed itself through the Irish language was slightly better, and was now raving in English, reciting Dylan Thomas. The neurologists saw him, and 'really, really' wanted us to do a lumbar puncture. I had decided against this when he came in because the procedure could be hazardous in an agitated and confused patient, but if they *really really* wanted a lumbar puncture, I told my registrar, they could take him over, an invitation they declined. No procedure is too hazardous for your colleagues to ask *you* to carry out.

An email from the senior speech and language therapist – to all users – told us that there was now a new vocabulary for dysphagia (swallowing problems) and that henceforth all hospital staff must use this nomenclature.

Over the years, I had fought a long war of attrition with the speech and language therapists. In acute hospitals, these therapists do not, as you might suppose, deal very much with speech and language problems; their main activity is assessment of swallowing. They were great enthusiasts for PEG feeding tubes, and often communicated this fervour to families, who then had to be talked down, sometimes with great difficulty. Since I was one of only two doctors in the ministry who routinely inserted PEG tubes, much of this difficult work came my way.

In many cases, it seemed to me that PEG feeding was more about fulfilling the complex emotional needs of relatives and staff than providing comfort for patients. I once gave a lecture – a grand round – on the subject, which I called 'Curb your enthusiasm'. Every speech and language therapist in the ministry sat stony-faced in the front row of the lecture hall.

A week later, the woman at the canteen checkout told me that I didn't have to pay for my lunch.

'Why, is it free today?' I asked.

'No, *she*—' (pointing to the woman before me in the queue) 'paid for it.'

'Why would she do that?'

'She said it was a random act of kindness.'

My benefactor wore the red top of a speech and language therapist.

A secret

Declan had attended my clinic, on and off, for many years, with a variety of ever-changing 'medically unexplained symptoms'. I listened intently to a lengthy exposition of his latest concerns. Carefully, hesitantly, I broached with him the possibility of psychological factors. Declan responded to this by telling me that he strongly suspected that all this was caused by food intolerances, and could I not do tests for these?

A couple of years before, I had attended a lecture by a liaison psychiatrist who specialised in treating patients with 'medically unexplained symptoms'. She explained, slowly and deliberately, as if she was teaching very small children, that once you demonstrated clearly to patients such as Declan the relationship between mind and body, between 'stressful life events' and their symptoms, they would achieve insight and would agree to – no, they would *embrace* – psychological treatments such as cognitive behavioural therapy. I liked this doctor but wondered if she practised in some parallel universe where the patients were as sweetly reasonable as she.

*

A middle-aged woman with Down syndrome, 'non-verbal', according to her carer. She thanked me by blowing a kiss.

A man wearing tinted spectacles. Tinted spectacles! They had all but disappeared, and encountering a wearer now made me nostalgic for the days when these spectacles were thought to be irrefutable evidence that the wearer's symptoms would be 'medically unexplained' or 'functional'. This man had heart-burn and acid reflux that did not respond to the maximum dose of acid-reducing medication. I sent him for oesophageal pH measurement, which would probably show that he did *not* have acid reflux. The hard bit would be imparting that news when he next came to my clinic. But that's how clinics worked: you had to bring the consultation to a conclusion; the next clinic would have to take care of itself.

It is a secret. Nobody tells the medical students that the out-patients and the GP surgeries are dominated by somatisers, the people with 'medically unexplained symptoms'. They are a small minority of the population, but vastly over-represented in the clinics. Over the years, I learned the skills of the long war of attrition; give a little territory now, but you win (or at least you are not overwhelmed) in the end. Wear them down, contain them, move them to other services. Buy time by booking tests with a long waiting list. Listen intently to everything they have to say; they will talk for as long as you can bear it, regardless of the crowded waiting room. Write down *everything*, because the stories often change: the woman whose life is intolerable today because of diarrhoea will turn up in three months saying that her bowels are fine, but this *pain* is so bad she has considered suicide.

Their bodies are corporeal Armageddons, sites of a never-ending battle between the forces of health and the vastly superior battalions of disease. Their battered immune systems are constantly assailed by toxins and foods. Patienthood is their occupation, their life's work. And, because they are human, they will eventually get something serious and die. More than a few greeted this news with an equanimity that hitherto had eluded them.

Doctors often resent somatisers because they drain their spirit; with each consultation they extract a little more of the soul. They resent them too because they tend to elbow the sick aside. I have spent far more time listening to the dietary concerns of people with abdominal bloating than I have spent attending to the needs of the dying. Sir William Osler was more forgiving: 'Deal gently then with this deliciously credulous old human nature in which we work, and restrain your indignation.'

As I drove home, my registrar phoned me about the Scottish woman with lung cancer. The biopsy confirmed cancer, but more worryingly, the official report of her CT scan said that the tumour was invading the pulmonary artery, with the risk of catastrophic, probably fatal, haemorrhage. She was desperate to go home. Was it safe, he asked, to let her? We were not going to do anything more; the oncologists had arranged to see her at their clinic. Let her go, I said, thinking that *safety* was no longer her priority.

That evening, I went to a retirement party. The retiring doctor had been at the ministry since 1993; we had known each other since the late 1980s when we both worked in Edinburgh. He had been the only emergency medicine consultant for his first five years at the ministry, during which time he was *permanently* on call. One Sunday afternoon during these lonely years, he reached crisis point. The emergency department waiting room was full; two junior doctors had phoned in sick; several unstable patients had come in after major trauma. My friend surveyed the packed waiting room. 'If there's anyone here who's not actually *dying*,' he addressed the crowd, 'would you ever fuck off?'

Silently, without protest, they rose as one to their feet, and meekly filed out.

The talker

The queue into the ministry's car park was already busy at 7.00 a.m. Security staff directed the traffic; women applied make-up while they sat waiting. Some came even earlier to bag a space, and then dozed for an hour in their cars.

⌒

The man suing us was still attending my colleague's clinic. I told her I would refuse to see a patient who was suing me. 'But he's a lovely man,' she said generously.

⌒

I gave my tutorial on 'Literature and Medicine'; one of the books on the reading list was Tolstoy's *The Death of Ivan Ilyich*. This book is often cited by palliative care doctors as a description of what Cicely Saunders* called 'total pain', meaning suffering that is not only physical, but also psychological and spiritual. I asked the group of twenty final-year students if anyone could name Tolstoy's most famous novel. After a long silence, a serious young man put his hand up and ventured: '*Crime and Punishment?*'

On my way to the tutorial, I passed the talker, who was holding forth in his preferred location, the intersection of two corridors. He had gathered an audience of three, who appeared to be hypnotised. When I finished the tutorial an hour later, he was *still* in position, but there were three new victims. I went to the canteen for lunch, and when I emerged thirty minutes later, the talker had not left; he was on to his *third* audience, now just two, laughing nervously, no doubt trying to conjure an excuse that would enable them to leave. The talker's usual themes were the extreme busyness of his clinic, the uselessness of senior management, and the personal lives of his colleagues. His indiscretion – which was legendary – half-attracted his listeners, but within five minutes they invariably felt trapped. He had a sorcerer's gift of immobilising them; desperate to flee, they were rooted to the spot by some malevolent power. The only escape was to be replaced by another human sacrifice.

* Dame Cicely Saunders (1918–2005) is regarded as the founder of the speciality of palliative care.

I went for a stroll around the cemetery near the ministry. A funeral was in progress: the priest had a big, peasant face; a woman wore sunglasses, even though the day was overcast – a touch of *The Sopranos*? At the far south-east end of the cemetery, along the wall of a workman's shed, there was a plot for unmemorialised children – orphans, stillbirths: 'Please pray for the babies buried here'. A toy duck hung from a tree, suspended by a noose of twine around its neck, almost as if it was a gibbet.

Walking back from the cemetery to the office, I met an old boss. We stopped to talk. I thought how much I liked him. His patients liked him too, even though they guessed he wasn't very bright. Perhaps they liked him for this very reason, and because he gave of himself. Other, more cerebral, physicians might have diagnosed and treated the patients more correctly, but they preferred him. He *liked* them, so they liked *him*. He was deaf to the bat-squeak of mockery, as enthusiastic in his mid-seventies as the day he graduated.

Wisdom and experience were no longer enough for the quotidian demands of the life clinical. Perhaps there is an intersection, sometime in the forties, where age and energy, enthusiasm and experience, meet in happy conjunction.

I recalled Michael, only a year ahead of me, but fully formed as a doctor by his mid-twenties. There was a balletic elegance, a gracefulness, in the way he examined patients; he rarely needed to repeat a manoeuvre. Did he get better as he got older? I never found out. An American-based professor of medicine – a local graduate – came home every year to recruit the brightest young doctors for his department. He took Michael out for a round of golf and offered him a job. I never heard of him again.

'What's this *mindfulness* they all keep talking about?' the surgeon-with-bottom asked me in the endoscopy unit. (Terence, head of health and wellbeing, had exhorted us all to 'practise mindfulness' in that week's wellbeing messages.)

I told him.

'Sure, that's the same as being a *dog*.'

A woman in an SUV drove out of the car park through the one-way entrance lane, nearly running me over. We made eye contact, her expression one of pure malice.

A *Festschrift*

Maddalena, my embryonic super-tanker, came with *both* parents to the outpatient clinic. I listened, for thirty minutes, to her father's theories on Maddalena's ill health: toxins, food intolerance, parasites, 'inflammation'. Maddalena sat silent, as impassive as a blancmange, as did her Irish mother. When I tried to make eye contact with her, she averted her gaze. How desperately I wanted to tell her: 'Your father is crazy. He is using you as a pawn in some game you and I will never understand. There is nothing wrong with you. Run away – now.'

A woman of sixty, wheelchair-bound by a neurodegenerative disease, complained of *intolerable* abdominal discomfort and bloating.

'I prayed to God that He might inspire you,' said her husband to me.

I suggested a non-absorbable antibiotic, often used for small intestinal bacterial overgrowth.* Although there was no reason why this woman should have such overgrowth, I felt under pressure to *do something*.

'But it won't kill the *good* bugs, will it?' she asked.

'No, only the *bad* ones,' I replied unconvincingly, as if antibiotics had some form of moral sensibility.

Distinguished academic doctors are sometimes given a *Festschrift*, a scientific symposium in their honour, 'a secular act of devotion'. I had been to one such event that went disastrously awry. The retiring doctor was one of the last of the NHS clinician-aristocrats, the only superior whose good opinion I had ever actively sought or valued. The symposium was graced by a Nobel laureate, who barely mentioned the man in whose honour we had gathered, concentrating instead on himself. The final speaker was allocated twenty minutes, but spoke for forty-five, on 'laser confocal endomicroscopy'. Two years later, I read this report in the *British Medical Journal*:

> An award-winning researcher who pioneered the use of laser confocal endomicroscopy to detect and treat early bowel cancer faked the results of a study published in the journal *Gut*, a General Medical Council panel was told last week.

---

* Small intestinal bacterial overgrowth means the presence of excess bacteria in the small intestine (which is normally almost sterile). This can cause chronic diarrhoea and malabsorption.

I searched the issue in vain for news of the Nobel laureate.

Some 'tributes' to distinguished colleagues are minor comic classics. Here is the Edinburgh-based physiologist Reggie Passmore's 1982 essay on his friend Sir Stanley Davidson (1894–1981), Professor of Medicine at the University of Edinburgh (1938–59) and author of the hugely popular text-book *Principles and Practice of Medicine* (commonly known as 'Davidson'):

> He was in no sense an intellectual and did not read widely. Unlike many professors, he was unafraid of displaying his ignorance by asking naïve questions. He was not a good writer by nature, but would spend endless time revising drafts of what he and others had written with an unerring eye for a clumsy phrase or a meaningless sentence. A cynical friend once remarked: 'Poor Stanley, he has only 500 words in his vocabulary, but he does know how to use them.' This legitimate exaggeration helps to explain why students loved his books so much.
>
> No account of Stanley Davidson would be complete without reference to money, a continuing preoccupation in both his private and public life. No Scot was ever more careful in spending sixpence. I used to be asked to bring a bottle of distilled water from the laboratory for his car batteries because the garage was now charging him too much. There are many similar stories.

I sat in on the senior house officers' appraisals. This was designed to monitor their progress, both professional and personal. One young woman was so obviously distressed the chairman offered to meet her on her own later. She hated the work and had failed her postgraduate exams. She stayed, she said, only to please her doctor father.

A Zambian doctor called Joseph came to the ministry in the 1980s to train in paediatrics. He struggled. 'You must remember', said the most senior doctor in that department, 'that Joseph is a long way from his *own parish*.' I was moved by this generosity of spirit.

Schwartz

I went to the Schwartz round* at lunchtime. This is an American import, 'an opportunity for healthcare staff to reflect on the emotional aspects of their work'. The small room was crowded and hot. There were three speakers: a nurse, a junior doctor and a clinical psychologist. The psychologist spoke last, pointedly scrolling her phone throughout the other talks. The nurse had worked in Africa, where, despite their poverty, the people radiated happiness. When she returned to Ireland,

---

* Ken Schwartz was an American lawyer who was diagnosed with incurable lung cancer in 1994 at the age of forty; he died less than a year later. During his treatment, he found that what mattered most to him were simple acts of kindness, acts that made 'the unbearable bearable'. Before his death, he left a legacy for the establishment of the Schwartz Center in Boston to foster compassion in health care. Schwartz himself laid down the rules for the rounds: they should be held in the middle of the day, preceded by a buffet lunch. A story is told by three or four people, but only one should be a doctor. The stories should last for a few minutes, with no formal presentations, and no applause. Latecomers are not admitted, and the round stops promptly at one hour. The discussion is led by a facilitator. There must be absolute confidentiality for both patients and staff.

she was appalled by how her patients – who had access to health care the Africans could only dream of – complained about *everything*. She had decided to return to Africa.

The junior doctor told a story about how he had found the courage to question the incorrect diagnosis of a more senior doctor, thereby saving a patient. The psychologist spoke about treating a cancer patient, and the bond she had formed with the patient and their family.

The event was facilitated by a tall, thin, nervous woman I did not recognise; she struggled to generate a discussion. Had she not been on a course, facilitated by a facilitator, for facilitators? 'Do any of these stories resonate?' she asked, with just a hint of desperation. An awkward silence followed. Eventually, a manager spoke about the primacy of a relative's intuition over the professional opinion of a doctor. 'You just *know* when your mother is not right,' he said with feeling. Many in the room nodded vigorously. His presence was proof of senior management's approval of this initiative; he had the Pharisee's nose for what was modish. Only three months before, a commissioned report – *Evaluation of the Introduction of Schwartz Rounds in Ireland* – concluded that these rounds made 'a significant contribution to staff engagement'.

The Schwartz rounds were an institutionalisation of what used to happen privately, between trusted friends, over a drink, but those days were over. I looked around the room, asking myself would I share my fears and my failures with *these* people? Could I divulge my error and neglect to the facilitator and the Pharisee manager? Would they help me achieve 'closure' on these troubles?

Eternity in hell will be filled with multidisciplinary team meetings and workshops. The fourth hierarchy of demons will be known as 'facilitators'. 'In hell', wrote the legal scholar Grant Gilmore, 'there will be nothing but law, and due process will be meticulously observed.'

⌒

An email was sent to all users on 'changes in dysphagia terminology':

> All staff involved in patient care, and the provision of food and beverages to patients with dysphagia will need to familiarise themselves with this framework. Representatives from Nutricia will be on the wards providing training.

I wondered how the ministry had allowed – indeed, actively encouraged – a commercial producer of 'nutritional supplements' to lead this Orwellian re-education of staff.

Food – once a source of comfort, sustenance and conviviality – had been medicalised, something that could be 'prescribed'. When the ministry opened, every ward had a little galley kitchen where the nurses made small, simple dishes – typically scrambled egg on toast – for those whose appetite had deserted them. This creaturely practice was banned for health and safety reasons, although I'm not sure what threat the preparation of scrambled eggs posed to safety. The frail, elderly, 'sarcopenic' people who constituted the majority of the ward patients were instead 'prescribed', at the behest of the dieticians, regular bottles of these nutritional supplements. The manufacturers sold this gloop to the hospital at a discount, but in 'the community' – as the world outside the ministry was now called – these supplements were expensive. The makers correctly anticipated that once a patient was prescribed the stuff in the ministry, they might well be given a prescription to continue when they were discharged. Heroin addicts – who tended to lose their appetite – were enthusiastic users, consuming the supplements as an alternative to food. It also freed up a lot of time in their busy days.

Although the ministry had become obsessed with 'nutrition', *food* had been increasingly neglected. Lunch trays were often placed in front of old people too sick to feed themselves in a ward too short of nurses who might spoon-feed them, in a world where relatives did not come in to help with this most simple of services. The ministry, unusually for a hospital of its size, prepared all the food on site, and, as hospital food goes, it wasn't bad. The bland, glutinous, but strangely moreish chicken curry served once a week in the canteen was so popular with staff that many (including me) looked forward to 'curry Tuesday'.

'A mental and physical *wreck*!'

News of the death of the long-retired professor; he was retired so long that his successor was now nearing retirement. Appointed in his mid-thirties, he was in post for thirty years. A devout churchgoer, a knight-member of an Irish Catholic fraternal organisation, the professor was at the zenith of his powers when the ministry opened in 1978. How he relished that power. We once clashed furiously at a public debate in the mid-1980s about the future of the medical profession, when he spoke for the consultants, and I for the junior doctors. 'Look at *him*,' he snarled, pointing at me, 'a mental and physical *wreck*!'

He was of that generation of clinical professors who saw their role as teachers and leaders, not generators of research grant income. Although he was an impressive and memorable clinical teacher, he was also a bully. I was shocked when, years after his retirement, I attended a black-tie event and heard him being booed by some of my contemporaries as he gave the after-dinner speech. How they hated him, never forgiving old humiliations.

I last saw him at the ill-fated launch of a book by one of his colleagues.* Now in his late eighties, the professor had been standing for some time for the author's over-lengthy speech, when he fainted, and crashed to the floor of the crowded gallery.† The first to his aid was a retired nurse who had been his ward sister for twenty years. Immediately behind her in the queue to assist was my brother, a geriatrician.

⌒

I carried out a gastroscopy on a woman who, after the procedure, was overcome by hysterical laughter. It reminded me of one of my professors at medical school, a man of demonic irritability, who once gave a lecture on the physiology of laughter, not an activity he devoted much time to – laughing, I mean, not lecturing. Earlier in his career, he had been medical officer of a steel company in Africa. One day, a man fell into the works furnace, dying instantly. His fellow workers stared down at his charred remains and burst into laughter. The professor's point was that laughter can be a physiological response to extreme stress and emotional trauma. John Lennon reacted to news of the death of his best friend, Stuart Sutcliffe, in 1962 in the

---

* Ill-fated, because the book received the worst review I have ever read. This daylight assassination was like coming upon a car crash with mangled, bleeding bodies. You wanted to look away but could not.

† This incident reminded me of the episode in *The Acceptance World* (the third novel in Anthony Powell's *A Dance to the Music of Time* sequence) when the public school housemaster, Le Bas, collapses at an annual dinner for the school's old boys at the Ritz, during an unsolicited (and very long) speech by Widmerpool. 'A sudden pang of impotent rage may even have contributed to other elements in bringing on his seizure.'

same manner. Inappropriate laughter, it is reported – although I have never witnessed it – can also be a rare symptom of brain-stem disease and injury; there is a growing literature on the neural pathways of laughter. My own suspicions about the origins of this phenomenon owed more to demonology than to neuroscience.

I had lunch with a friend, a doctor in another department. Her colleagues were already squabbling, with more than three months to go, over the 'on-call' for Christmas and the New Year. There are two sure ways – apart from marriage – of *really* getting to know people: play football with them, *qua* Camus, or share an on-call rota.

An elderly man passed me on the main corridor; he looked familiar. Yes, it was *him,* the grand gynaecologist. I thought he was dead. The surgeon-with-bottom once told me a story about him. He happened to mention to the grand gynaecologist that he was moving house. The gynaecologist asked who was doing the moving? The surgeon gave the name of a local removals firm. 'No, no,' smiled the gynaecologist indulgently, 'I meant who is moving your *claret?*'

'Very big person in medicine, yes?'

The first patient at the clinic that morning was a French-woman, whom I had fully investigated for abdominal pain, finding no cause. She had phoned her brother, a wealthy businessman, who put her in contact with a friend of his, a professor in Paris ('very big person in medicine, yes?'). She phoned this professor, who immediately diagnosed pancreatic insufficiency.* My patient bought pancreatic enzyme capsules while on holiday at home, and now pronounced herself cured.

'That's very good,' I said.

'But why do *you* not diagnose this?'

I tried to explain that her pancreas was normal on her CT scan, that this was a disease of alcoholics (she was teetotal), but this made no impression on her. Her dramatic recovery demonstrated both the remarkable power of the placebo as

---

* A condition characterised by deficiency of pancreatic digestive enzymes, leading to malabsorption of fat and some vitamins. Alcohol-related chronic pancreatitis is the most common cause.

well as the importance of the prescribing doctor's status. I was not, she clearly felt, a 'very big person in medicine'.

When I called the next patient, a woman of seventy-four, from the waiting room, her phone rang with a deafening ringtone.

'I read an article about your book,' she said, 'the one about death.'

'Oh, really?'

'You've got it *right*, boy!'

A man of seventy was dressed like a teenager, wearing a track-suit, baseball hat and trainers. He had attended my clinic for years, being a 'martyr' to his bowels.

'How are things?' I ventured cautiously.

'Terrible.'

'Terrible in what way?'

'Five days I'm constipated, then two days I've got diarrhoea. The wind is unbearable. Foul-smelling. You wouldn't believe it.'

His colonoscopy showed some diverticulitis,* generally harmless, and very common in the over-seventies.

'Why can't you send me for an operation to remove the diverticulitis?'

'Because that wouldn't help your bowels or your wind.'

He looked disappointed. I changed the subject.

* Diverticula are small pouches in the lining of the colon, which become more common with age. Most people do not have symptoms.

'Still smoking twenty a day?'

'I'm going to see a hypnotist,' he said, 'but I'm waiting for the social welfare to pay for it.'

'How much does the hypnotist charge?'

'Ninety-nine euro.'

'Why not a hundred?'

'Ninety-nine sounds cheaper.'

Two patients were sent by their GPs to the clinic for 'screening' colonoscopy because they had 'a family history of colon cancer'. I was able to find their relatives' biopsy results on the laboratory digital IT system; both did indeed have cancer, but neither had *colon* cancer.

At the entrance to the canteen, I passed a desk festooned with information aimed at raising awareness of malnutrition in hospital patients. This was sponsored by Nutricia, manufacturer of nutritional supplements, and now also a provider of training for health professionals on dysphagia terminology. I mentioned to the dietician who was manning this stall that they were in competition for my awareness with 'infection prevention week'. 'But you need to be well nourished to fight infection,' she countered cheerfully. 'Would you like a pen?' The pen bore the logo 'Nutricia'.

My senior house officer told me that a patient under another medical team had died overnight. The patient's consultant, she said approvingly, 'was *very* upset'. Such displays of emotion were increasingly expected of doctors.

'No regrets?'

I handed my letter of resignation to the chief executive's personal assistant this morning. This job, so difficult to obtain, I now almost casually handed back. Few wanted these posts now, but twenty years ago the competition was intense. Highly qualified doctors who had overcome every hurdle and jumped through every hoop found themselves, after a few months, in Donie's office in Purchasing, being told that there was no money for new equipment this year. No wonder so many of them became ravenous beasts, red in tooth and claw.

The first year back at the ministry (2001–2) was hard. I inherited a service so moribund that I wondered if it could ever be revived. I had no office; the endoscopy 'unit' was two tiny rooms in the outpatients; I was charged with developing a therapeutic endoscopy service, but there was no equipment; when I tried to introduce new procedures, I was told: 'This is how we've always done it here.'

My first week – the days running up to 9/11 – was comically, catastrophically, bad. A patient had a serious complication – a colonic perforation – after my very first endoscopy list.

⌒

The grand round was on malnutrition, sponsored, inevitably, by Nutricia, who paid for the coffee and sandwiches. A physician from another hospital in the city came in late and sat next to me. She scrolled on her phone throughout the lecture, looking up occasionally, not at the screen, but to see who else was there in the room.

A nervous dietician, speaking with a high-rising Australian intonation, presented the case of a woman with metastatic breast cancer, who, not surprisingly, had lost weight. The dietician explained how she calculated this patient's nutritional deficit and requirements; the treatment, predictably, was nutritional supplements of the kind manufactured by Nutricia.

A specialist in acute medicine concluded the meeting by speaking about the latest guidelines from the European society for parenteral and enteral nutrition. These guidelines, he said pompously, were 'consensus-driven'. 'Consensus', I reflected, occupied the lowest position in the hierarchy of medical evidence.

⌒

A letter from the radiation specialist, informing me that Daithi, the man with the cancer-induced high blood calcium, and the subject of so much squabbling, had died, less than two weeks after his admission. The music had finally stopped; the parcel was empty.

To the outpatients, where the first patient was an anorexic girl, gum-chewing, sullen, described in a recent letter by a junior doctor from another department as 'lovely'. Having reached sixteen, she was discharged by the child and adolescent mental health service; her mother told me she might have to wait for a year to transfer to the adult service. She was sent to me with 'constipation', a near universal symptom of this disease; I wondered if the GP just wanted someone, *anyone*, to share the pain.

There was an ever-increasing pressure in the ministry to reconfigure anorexia as a purely *nutritional* problem; I had once refused to be involved in 'involuntary' treatment, meaning force-feeding. My view on this – that it was barbaric, unethical, and probably futile – was not shared by the psychiatrists. I understood their nervousness: severe anorexia has a high mortality rate; they did not want dead bodies in their unit. They sent the refractory, end-stage anorexics instead to my colleague, who was steadily accumulating the largest collection of super-tanker patients in the ministry. His even temper and lack of vanity suited him for this responsibility, but I wondered what monsters were being created.

I reviewed a man with colitis who had been on an immuno-suppressive drug for nine years. I went over his case notes; it had been started for the flimsiest of reasons and the pre-scription was renewed every six months without reviewing the need for its continuation. Luckily, he did not question me closely when I told him he could stop it. What would I have said? That the doctor who put you on this is lazy and thoughtless?

⌒

The medical school sent an email, which read like a spoof from Myles na Gopaleen's (Flann O'Brien) *Cruiskeen Lawn* column in *The Irish Times*, advertising a talk by Professor Dr Clemens Kunz. He had trained, the email said, with Professor Egge of Bonn University, 'one of the pioneers in human milk oligosaccharides'.

⌒

As I was about to start my car to drive home, someone knocked on my window.

'I hear you're leaving,' said a colleague. 'My wife told me.'

His wife was also a doctor at the ministry. I handed in my resignation only that morning; how did she find out so quickly? Did she have a mole in the chief executive's office? I had to concede that this was impressive. What an intelligence agent she would have made.

'No regrets?'

'None.'

'There's the dead, and
the dead dead'

I began the mournful task of sorting through my office contents. This is how it ends – in details, minor details.

It being a fine day, I went for a lunchtime walk to the cemetery. I found the neglected grave of one Raymond de Vericour. The headstone featured a portrait (in bas-relief) of this noble-looking man. I looked him up when I returned to the office: he was a Frenchman, professor of modern languages at the university (then called Queen's College Cork) from 1849 to 1879 and a biographer of Dante. 'There's the dead,' a neighbour once told me, 'and the dead dead.' Who now prays at the grave of Raymond de Vericour?

The clinic weighing scales reads in kilograms. Every other patient asks: 'What's that in stones?'

'I don't know,' I always say, 'it reads in kilos.'

My first outpatient that day was a well-groomed, courteous Argentinian woman in her mid-forties. I asked what brought her to Ireland.

'I am a missionary.'

'Really? What is your faith?'

She smiled. 'Christian, of course.' Did she not know that this city, in my boyhood a place of Redemptorist Lenten retreats and Corpus Christi processions that stopped traffic, once regarded itself as a citadel of the Faith? Did she not know that this city once sent priests, nuns and brothers all over the world? Did she not know that St Joseph's apostolic college – a stone's throw from this clinic – once trained missionary priests? Did she not know that Raymond de Vericour was nearly dismissed by the university because he had written a book* thought to be anti-Catholic in sentiment? Did she not know that her ministry here was a bizarre historical reversal?

*

* *An Historical Analysis of Christian Civilisation* (1850), in which de Vericour wrote: 'Nothing satisfactory is really known about the Bishop of Rome's assuming pontifical authority.' Hard to imagine such a book causing a scandal now, but it did in 1850, and Vericour was suspended by the university's administration; Cardinal Paul Cullen, the Archbishop of Armagh, called him 'a French infidel'. De Vericour successfully appealed on the technical grounds that the non-denominational charter of the university required neutrality on religious issues in the classroom only.

A bald man with a ponytail was worried about candida,* or 'can-deeda', as those stricken by this concern pronounce it. I thought 'can-deeda' had gone the way of such 1980s' passing phenomena as tinted spectacles and foam neck-collars, but no, it clung on, like some religious cult, immune to scientific evidence and new, more fashionable ailments.

'I was exposed to someone with a fungal infection,' he explained.

'Hmm...' I answered, having long ago learned that questioning this delusion was futile.

'It's giving me throat mucus, burning mouth and itchy anus.'

---

* A fungal infection that commonly affects the oral cavity and vagina ('thrush'). 'Invasive' candidiasis, where there is infection of internal organs such as the oesophagus, occurs rarely, mainly in people with compromised immunity, typically those with HIV/AIDS. Beginning in the 1980s, many people began to believe that candida caused irritable bowel syndrome and chronic fatigue; this belief was encouraged by many complementary and alternative medicine (CAM) practitioners. I always explained to patients who expressed this concern that yes, candida *did* sometimes cause 'deep' infection in the digestive system, but *only* in people with immune deficiency. These efforts at reassurance were generally fruitless; the patients would often move on to CAM practitioners who would generally confirm the diagnosis of candida (by various bizarre 'tests') and prescribe some form of treatment, which they claimed was 'antifungal'.

By the 2000s, 'candida' had become less fashionable, and its preeminent place as the concern of patients with 'medically unexplained symptoms' was gradually overtaken by food intolerance. I cannot quite explain this fading away. Perhaps 'candida' was too *generic* as a diagnosis: lots of people seemed to be diagnosed with it, whereas with food intolerance, there was an infinite number of possible permutations, a way for the patient to have a *unique* affliction: 'I am intolerant to wheat, citrus and asparagus, but my son is intolerant to lactose, beetroot and all legumes.' There remains, however, a confluence where food intolerance and candida meet: some CAM therapists claim that a diet that eliminates sugar, alcohol, gluten and dairy 'cures' candida.

Taking to the bed

The first patient I saw on the ward round was a woman of thirty-five, raving and confabulating, in a side room, watched over by a nervous 'special', a large, heavily tattooed man. A homeless alcoholic, she had fallen over drunk in the street, banged her head, and sustained bilateral subdural brain haemorrhages (haematomas). The neurosurgeons drained the haematomas, but she had not recovered. Random words spilled from her mouth; she pointed repeatedly at her belly. The brain injury had destroyed her powers of both comprehension and expression. I examined her with great difficulty. Is this what they meant by 'a fate worse than death'?

Little Tommy was in a side room on a surgical ward. As usual, his father was with him. I had known Little Tommy since he was a child; he was now twenty-four and had spent much of his life in the ministry. He had been dealt a poor genetic hand, with a combination of two rare diseases, one afflicting the liver, the other the lungs. As usual, I told him that the *one* important thing he could do for himself was to give up smoking. As usual, Little Tommy said: 'I know, but it's very hard to give up the fags.' As usual, I said: 'I know, Tommy, I know.'

Little Tommy was no better; his father told me how fed up and frustrated they both were. Tommy, his face moon-shaped and his tattooed arms wasted from years of steroids (taken for his liver condition), sobbed quietly. His liver disease was now advanced; we regularly drained fluid (ascites) from his abdomen, but it quickly reaccumulated. We would have to consider liver transplantation, but his chronic lung disease might be an impediment. I phoned one of the consultants at the national liver unit in Dublin, who agreed that he would arrange to transfer Little Tommy to their unit for 'a full assessment'.

Gary was in the medical short-stay unit with a bad pneumonia. A few years before, he had exchanged heroin for a combination of methadone and alcohol, but the alcohol – helped by the hepatitis C he had contracted from his needle use – gave him liver cirrhosis. Three weeks before, Gary had found his partner dead in bed. This prompted him to give heroin one last chance.

Back on my 'home' ward, a woman of seventy-one, who looked ninety-one, had taken to the bed for unknown reasons. I started with the basics of history and physical examination, which was difficult because she was irritable and uncooperative, then looked at her blood tests and X-rays. I could find no medical reason why she should be bed-bound; perhaps it was simply her preferred environment. There is a long, not entirely dishonourable, tradition of 'taking to the bed' in Ireland; only recently has this form of social withdrawal been reconfigured as a *medical* problem. Martha, the ward's clinical nurse manager, had spoken to her husband, concluding that he was 'simple'; he did confirm, however, that his wife had been in bed for 'about a year'.

We assume that because someone is in hospital, *in a bed*, that they must be *sick*. Most are, but sometimes – like this patient – they were there because no one could think of any other solution to their existential problem. Declaring that a patient was *not sick* was quite a brave 'diagnosis' for a doctor to make, but it was one I often made, usually after waiting for a few days, just in case something I had missed declared itself. I had watched this woman for the obligatory few days, and nothing changed.

Hers was now a 'placement' problem: the discharge co-ordinator would be the most important person in her management. She would eventually go to a nursing home, whenever a vacancy could be found in one, and when her family had completed the (for some) difficult forms. This might take many weeks – even months – during which it was highly likely that this woman would succumb to some hospital-acquired ('nosocomial') infection or fall out of bed. Elderly patients in the ministry were for ever falling out of bed, sometimes sustaining serious injuries, such as a broken hip. One of the commonest night-time calls to the most junior doctors (interns) is to see a patient who has 'fallen out of bed'.

*

A super-tanker patient with chronic abdominal pain asked me, only half-seriously: 'You *don't* have a magic wand?'

When first encountering a liver patient, the most important question was this: was there any possibility, however remote, that this patient might get transplanted? In most, the answer was 'no', and the emphasis of treatment gradually, inexorably, went down the 'palliative path'. The notes on two liver patients finally arrived on the ward two days after their admission. One woman had multiple liver tumours, which I did not know when I had first seen her. Neither did she.

⌒

World Stroke Day. A stroke nurse sat at a table by the ministry's main entrance, wearing a red T-shirt bearing the admonishment 'Don't be the 1 in 4' – one in four people will have a stroke during their lifetime.* A sad, semi-deflated red balloon bearing the same slogan was taped to the desk.

Stroke had done well lately in the My Disease Is Better Than Your Disease competition, far better than liver disease. Stroke had its own ward in the ministry now; it had specialist

---

* I thought they could have come up with a more original slogan: One in Four is also an Irish charity that assists adults who have experienced childhood sexual abuse. These days there are so many charities and patient support groups, they *share* slogans. Even the gimmicks are shared. The ice-bucket challenge – where willing good sports are doused in cold water to raise awareness of motor neurone disease – was later hijacked by the Macmillan cancer campaign.

nurses and its slogan and red balloons. There was no World Alcoholic Liver Disease Day, however; no famous patient advocates, no catchy slogan, no balloons. I consoled myself that at least I did not have to sit at a desk handing out quizzes and pens.

At the journal club, a drug rep supplied coffee and muffins and gave a ten-minute talk on her product. She winked, vulgarly and knowingly, at the male registrar who organised the meeting.

My inner child

At the outpatients, I began with a man in his sixties, who had 'an awful time with the allergies'.

'What are you allergic to?' I asked.

'Gluten and milk.'

'Who diagnosed that?'

'A Chinese man in the shopping centre.'

'How did he make the diagnosis?'

'He took one of my hairs.'

A woman with chronic abdominal pain, whose investigations were all normal.

'I'm just wondering if I might have – what's it called? – post something.'

'Post-traumatic stress disorder?'

'That's the one. My daughter says I might have it.'

'Why does she say that?'

'My son hung himself. I found him.'

⁓

A nurse told me she was going to contribute to the next Schwartz round.

'What are you going to talk about?' I asked.

'My inner child.'

⁓

I visited my mother on the trauma ward; she was recovering there after surgery to repair a broken hip. I watched the scene in the opposite bed. A man was trying to spoon-feed an old woman, his mother, presumably. She shook her head; he persisted, as if she were a difficult toddler. The man was a hunchback. I left the room while my mother was being toileted. The hunchback came out too, to make a phone call: 'She's starving to death,' he told his interlocutor. 'She'll never get better if she doesn't eat.'

I recalled the hunchback surgeon. In the mid-1980s, when he retired from his NHS consultant post in Birmingham, he came to work in the ministry as a locum chest surgeon.* He would have been then in his late sixties. He treated everyone – patients, nurses and junior doctors – with an antique

* He took over from a fearsome man, described thus in his *Irish Times* obituary: 'He had a most imposing appearance – a larger than life figure, well over 6 ft, carefully groomed, broad shouldered with trademark centre parting of his huge head of hair. Nothing but the best was good enough for his patients. He was dogmatic, ruthless, not particularly popular with colleagues and often rubbed people up the wrong way.'

courtesy. His handsome face was lean and aristocratic; his hair was snow-white. The nurses adored him; it was not pity, but *tenderness*. He returned to England when a substantive consultant was eventually appointed; he worked into his late eighties as a hospice volunteer.

The Lord Mayor of the city – a hunchback – visited my school, sometime in the mid-1970s; three boys, gathered at the back of the school hall, mocked this man's deformity. A decade later, Gérard Depardieu played the eponymous hunchback in *Jean de Florette*. When a storm ruins his crop, he looks up at the skies and shouts at God: 'I'm a hunchback! Have you forgotten that? Do you think it's easy?'

The man they couldn't hang

My first patient on that day's ward round was a man in his forties in an extra bed – 'extra' meant the bed should *not* be there – on the corridor in the medical short-stay unit. He used a lot of medical jargon, mainly to let me know that he was a pharmacist. His case notes documented multiple admissions with gastrointestinal bleeding. I immediately suspected him of being addicted to Nurofen® Plus.* I had seen several patients with this dependence, one of whom had died.

To the intensive care unit to see Dan, a new admission. He had been an inpatient for a prolonged period three years before, spending thirteen months in the ministry.

---

* This is an over-the-counter medication, a combination of codeine (an opiate) and ibuprofen (an anti-inflammatory). Users become addicted to the codeine, requiring ever-increasing doses; unfortunately, this means they also consume ever-increasing doses of the ibuprofen, causing stomach ulcers and bleeding. Amazingly, it remains non-prescription.

An alcoholic, he somehow survived a series of mainly liver-related catastrophes. I joked with him then that he was 'the man they couldn't hang', a title in which he took some pride. In the years since then, Dan had no contact with the ministry. His ex-wife told me that he had spent that time watching TV and drinking the cheapest supermarket lager he could find. Now Dan had pneumonia, for which he required ventilation. The intensive care unit doctors were amazed by his recovery; I was not surprised.

The woman with multiple liver tumours was seen by an oncologist who requested yet another CT scan, which now showed a blood clot in a vein in her groin. My registrar was all for getting the radiologists to insert a caval filter,* to prevent the clot travelling to the lungs; it occurred to me that this would not be the worst way for her to die.

A woman in her forties was admitted directly from the endoscopy unit. She had come in as a day case for a colonoscopy, performed by one of my colleagues. When she was told that this was normal, she howled uncontrollably, refusing to go home. The only means of mollifying her was to admit her as an inpatient, with a promise from my colleague that he wouldn't discharge her until 'a definite diagnosis' had been reached. What would they put in the admission note as

* Mechanical filters placed in the inferior vena cava, the main vein of the abdomen and lower limbs, which drains into the heart. These filters block blood clots from migrating to the lungs (pulmonary embolism).

'presenting complaint'? Acute disappointment? Unbearable cognitive dissonance?

The Russian man with alcohol-induced seizures had recovered enough to complain: 'They have taken my papers.'

'What papers?' I asked.

'Passport and medical card.'

How John le Carré, I thought, 'papers'.

⌒

A few people who worked at the ministry when I was a house officer in the mid-1980s were still there, thirty-seven years later, as I neared retirement. They included Dinny in the mortuary, and Billy who fixed wheels. It was amazing how many things were attached to wheels, and how often these wheels broke. There was enough wheel-related work in the ministry to keep Billy busy; he had been fixing wheels since the ministry opened. He took some pride in this work, often wearing a T-shirt that proclaimed: 'I'm Billy, and I fix wheels'.

⌒

As if my bad eye and arthritic hands weren't enough, I was now getting regular, unexplained nosebleeds. These bleeds often occurred at the most inopportune times – during clinic, or when I was endoscoping.

'It just pays the bills'

Dan, the man they couldn't hang, had a big stomach bleed. I went over to the intensive care unit to see him; he was not well: pale, clammy, low blood pressure. He needed an urgent endoscopy, which a colleague generously agreed to do since I had to go back to clinic. My registrar told me that the pharmacist was 'creating havoc' in the medical short-stay unit. I would deal with him tomorrow, I said. I walked back down the crowded, damp, oppressive corridor, past the disabled folk waiting in the foyer near the front entrance for cars and taxis to collect them, through the wheezy huddle of smokers, and in heavy rain to the clinic building.

⌒

At the clinic, I saw an eighty-two-year-old man who had survived lung cancer.

'Were you a big smoker?' I asked.

'I never smoked a fag in my life,' he laughed, 'but long 'go the card players filled our house with smoke.'

A Polish woman was sent for investigation of anaemia. Although she had lived in Ireland for fifteen years, she was not confident with her English; her teenage son came in to help. We were supposed to use professional interpreters, but very often the GP's referral letter didn't mention any language barrier, and when the patients turned up at clinic, it was hard to turn them away and rebook another appointment with an interpreter. It was when I had to ask this woman, through her son, if she had heavy periods (the most likely cause of her anaemia) that I realised that this ban on family members as interpreters might, after all, be correct. The boy did not look embarrassed.

When I did my ward round the next day, Dan was stable; his endoscopy did not show any source of bleeding. I spoke to his ex-wife in the tiny, windowless room in the unit reserved for difficult conversations. She agreed with alacrity when I recommended that should Dan deteriorate further, our focus would be on 'comfort'. Their children, who were scattered all over the world, would, she assured me, agree.

The pharmacist who had been creating 'havoc' was now placated by the prescription of an opiate. His equanimity restored, he asked to go home. I funked the question about Nurofen® Plus. I told myself that he would deny it and be mortally offended, so I had saved myself unnecessary conflict; I didn't entirely convince myself.

I saw Little Tommy just as the ambulance driver was collecting him for his journey to the liver unit in Dublin. He told me he was terrified that he would be in hospital for Christmas. 'I just want to be at home with my family.'

⁓

I met a fellow consultant for coffee. I told him I had handed in my notice. His envy was palpable. 'I get no enjoyment out of this. It just pays the bills.'

⁓

I took a call from an old friend, now working in the north of England; we had trained together in the early 1990s at a grand old NHS teaching hospital. He wanted a favour: namely that I would take on a patient, a 'friend of a friend'. We talked for a while, catching up with each other's lives. He reminded me that I had once told him, when in the throes of some personal difficulty: 'You know when you're standing on the platform at a railway station? You don't expect the train to hit you, but that's what happened to me.' I had no recollection of saying this, but thought it a stylish remark.

'Welcome, Sister Death'

Dan, the man they couldn't hang, bled again during the night. There was a new duty consultant for the intensive care unit, who wanted a surgical opinion before committing ourselves irrevocably to 'comfort measures'. The duty consultants changed every few days; they sometimes took very differing views on the discontinuation of active treatment. Even though the name on the patient's sticker was *mine*, the intensive care unit consultants (all anaesthetists or intensivists) did most of the work and took the lead in decision-making. It took several phone calls to establish which surgeon was on call that day. The switchboard put me through to one who told me he was away at a conference, and that another was covering for him. I phoned this second surgeon, going straight to voicemail. He phoned back to say no, he wasn't on call, but he knew who was. The third surgeon was scrubbed in theatre when I called but phoned back ten minutes later and agreed to see Dan that evening.

My secretary left a message asking me to phone a GP who was 'very worried' about a patient with a high blood iron.* This did not strike me as an urgent problem, but I phoned anyway. The voice message informed me that the surgery was now closed. Driving out of the hospital, I spotted this same GP, lying on the lawn in front of the hospital, engaged in highly athletic stretching exercises. Her surgery was in a village sixty miles away, but she lived here in the city, commuting daily. As I drove past, she stood up and power-walked off, her short legs propelled by ski poles.

My mother was discharged back to her nursing home. She would miss, she told me, the ward nurses and the 'goings on'. Nurses were far more important to the patients than doctors, who appeared fleetingly. A kind nurse made all the difference to this sick, frightened old woman.

Good doctors (and good nurses) are self-effacing, humble, endlessly patient, full of common sense, constitutionally incapable of boredom. However, eminent and influential doctors – 'key opinion leaders' – are usually vain, arrogant, impatient and ambitious. A good doctor, in Auden's† phrase,

---

* A high level of iron in the blood is often caused by haemochromatosis, a hereditary condition where there is excessive absorption into the blood-stream of dietary iron. This disease is common in Ireland, where more than 1 per cent of the population is genetically predisposed. If untreated, it can lead to diabetes, liver cirrhosis and arthritis.

† Auden would have known a bit about doctoring; his father, George Augustus Auden, was physician at York County Hospital, and later professor of public health at the University of Birmingham.

should be broad-rumped, partridge plump, and not *too* clever.

⌒

This was both World Quality Day *and* World Diabetes Day. To mark the day, a diabetes nurse specialist had set up a stall in the canteen offering free blood glucose tests. She told me that to get the blood test, I would first have to do the diabetes quiz.

⌒

An email announced the 'digital academy forum'. This academy 'will train digital leaders who will deliver more cost-effective and better health services for Irish citizens'. I looked up the website: the new strategy was called 'stay left, shift left'. I was not quite sure what this meant, but, helpfully, they gave an example: 'a cloud-based solution to prevent diabetic foot ulcers'. Individuals with diabetes would weigh themselves daily; the 'smart' scales would take a picture and measure the temperature of the foot, 'sending this to a cloud for analysis by health professionals'. Where, I wondered, would these professionals *be*? Would there be designated digital centres where 'health professionals' looked at pictures of *feet*?

⌒

In the cemetery there is a Franciscan plot, with a plaque proclaiming: 'Welcome, Sister Death'. I thought this odd, for 'Death' is usually portrayed as male – the Grim Reaper, the figure in Bergman's *The Seventh Seal*, even Brad Pitt in *Meet Joe Black*.

One of the last citadels of male privilege had been breached. The porter covering endoscopy today was a young woman.

'*Fucking* way!'

I was fluish and out of sorts; not quite sick enough to be at home in bed, but just enough to feel miserable. On my way in, I met a colleague who had survived cancer. 'For a doctor to take a day off sick,' she said, 'you have to be *completely* incapacitated.'

Maddalena – the teenage girl with the overbearing father – was my first outpatient. The father came in to see me alone, leaving Maddalena temporarily in the waiting room. She, he maintained, must have cryptosporidiosis.* He had heard of a lot of people in the west of Ireland getting it from contaminated mains water. I logged on to the laboratory system; Maddalena's GP had sent three stool samples, all of which were negative for cryptosporidiosis.

* Cryptosporidiosis is a parasitic infection that can cause watery diarrhoea and persistent cough.

'You are sure?' the father asked with a pained expression.

'Quite sure. Why don't you bring Maddalena in?'

Maddalena came in, sat beside her father, and looked at the floor.

'Maddalena, how did you get on with that medication I gave you?'

Before she could speak, her father interjected: 'We read about that medication. It has lactose. Maddalena, she is allergic to lactose.'

When they eventually left, I pondered on the failure of the system, myself included, to challenge this man. Later that day, I phoned Maddalena's GP. I told her that although I didn't think that this was a case of Munchausen's syndrome by proxy, there was, nevertheless, something deeply suspicious going on, something I couldn't quite give a diagnostic *label* to: co-dependence? *Folie à deux*?

'Thank God,' she said, 'I thought I was the only one.'

We discussed what we should do. Social workers and psychiatrists had already been involved; what could *we* do? We sadly agreed that the most we could aim for was to *contain* the problem, to stop it getting worse.

I started my round in the emergency department. The first patient was an enormous Latvian woman with liver failure. She was deeply jaundiced; the skin over her distended belly was thick and puckered like orange peel. Her husband told me that they had been to the national liver unit in Dublin the week before. I phoned a consultant there, who agreed to take her. She would die, but it was better that she did so in a liver unit. Better that *they* turned her down for a transplant, not me.

Dan, the man they couldn't hang, was now stable enough to be discharged from the intensive care unit to the ward. The surgeon had prescribed a medication that appeared to be working miraculously well, because Dan had no further bleeding. I felt mildly ashamed that *I* had not thought of this – physicians are supposed to come up with these suggestions about new drugs, not *surgeons*.

In the queue for lunch at the canteen, a medical student, a bearded boy of twenty, was talking loudly enough for the whole line to hear. Wearing a purple scrubs top, he was all swagger as he described for his audience of fellow students his morning in the operating theatre. Why doesn't he just shut up? I thought; he knows *nothing*. And then it occurred to me that I was just like him when I was twenty. How we cringe, with age, to recall the thoughtless loutishness of youth.

But there was something qualitatively different about this boy's braggadocio, something of the *zeitgeist* about it. Television has been extraordinarily influential on people's conversation and behaviour. In *The Great War and Modern Memory*, the American literary scholar Paul Fussell argued that the First World War made irony the defining attribute of Western culture in the twentieth century; television produced a change in human perception and behaviour that was just as profound. When *The West Wing* introduced walking-and-talking – to show how busy the characters were – quite ordinary people began to behave in this presentational fashion. Just after the TV hospital drama *ER* started in the early 1990s, one of my fellow registrars took to wearing a pale-blue scrubs top (the rest of us were still in white coats) and tilting his head – just like George Clooney – to signal that he was listening intently. Then *Scrubs* arrived in the noughties, and an entire generation of medical students and junior doctors started to believe that hospitals were intrinsically funny.

On the way back to my office, I happened to be walking behind two female medical students, both Asian-Canadian.

'I'm like, you're fucking *joking*?' said one.

'No fucking way!'

'*Fucking* way!'

'Round early and round
a second time'

An email from the ministry's chief executive stated, with a firm grasp of the obvious, that there was 'a mismatch between capacity and demand'. He urged the consultants to 'round early and round a second time': that is, to carry out *two* ward rounds every day, seeing the *same* patients. Did he truly believe that some of them would have improved sufficiently in the interval between these rounds to be discharged? Or – more likely – was this exhortation merely a compulsory, centrally mandated tick-box component of the so-called 'escalation policy'?

~

The first outpatient was a young woman with irritable bowel syndrome, of the diarrhoea-predominant variety.* I looked

---

* There are four subtypes of irritable bowel syndrome (IBS): diarrhoea-

up her blood tests on the laboratory system; there were 1,240.

A man in his thirties, a lawyer. I had investigated him a few years before, diagnosing irritable bowel syndrome. This was triggered by the breakup of his marriage; he had been distressed enough then to attempt suicide. He told me that he had started a gluten-free diet and was now 'cured'. Although 'cured', he wanted a *formal* diagnosis of gluten sensitivity: 'It's important for me psychologically.' We had a long discussion; he probed carefully with a series of Jesuitical questions.

'Why didn't you pick up my gluten sensitivity three years ago?'

'I did blood tests and a biopsy. They were normal.'

'Could I be gluten-sensitive, but not coeliac?'

'If you're better on a gluten-free diet, then why not just stay on it?'

'I've read that a gluten-free diet can increase the risk of diabetes and heart disease. I want a *proper* diagnosis. Can't you do further tests?'

'You'd have to have what's called oral provocation testing.*

---

predominant; constipation-predominant; alternating diarrhoea and constipation, and bloating-predominant. This is known as the Rome classification, after the conference held there in 1994, which established orthodoxy within the global church of IBS researchers, just as the Council of Nicaea led to uniform Christian doctrine. These 'consensus' conferences are always held in congenial locations.

* Foods suspected of causing intolerance are disguised in capsules. Ideally, the test should be placebo-controlled and 'double-blind', i.e., neither the patient nor the doctor knows which capsule contains the 'offending' food. The patient is asked to report any symptoms on a visual analogue scale.

We can't do that here. And even if we could, I have reservations about that test.'

'What reservations?'

'That it's not really scientific.'

I was rescued from this interrogation by a call from a consultant at the national liver unit about Little Tommy.

'Forgive me, I have to take this. I'm on call,' I lied to the gluten-sensitive lawyer.

'We're not going to transplant Tommy,' the liver specialist said.

He explained that during their 'intensive pre-transplant work-up' they had discovered that Little Tommy's lung disease was more advanced than we had thought, that it had led to significant damage to his heart. If Tommy *were* to be transplanted, he would require not only a new liver, but a lung *and* heart transplant also. He would have to go to the UK for this, he said, and there was no guarantee that he would be accepted. They had discussed all this with Little Tommy; he told them that he didn't want a transplant, that he just wanted to be at home for Christmas. They were going to send Little Tommy back to the ministry.

I resumed my conversation with the lawyer, but it was difficult to give him my attention – or, indeed, my sympathy – when all I could think of was Little Tommy.

This test is so laborious that, apart from private food allergists who cater for the rich, it is almost exclusively used by researchers in clinical trials.

Over coffee, I leafed through a 1935 edition of Hamilton Bailey's* *Demonstrations of Physical Signs in Clinical Surgery*; I found it in the €2 pile at a second-hand bookshop in Macroom, a small market town west of Cork city. The book, first published in 1927, was still in print (and widely read) when I was a student. The photographic illustrations were grotesque; the subjects were often naked, easily identifiable, with extreme examples of their disease. I should lend my copy, I thought, to my gluten-sensitive lawyer.

⌣

* Bailey's biographer, Adrian Marston (himself a surgeon), wrote: 'He studied and recorded the diseased human body with immense care but was never a "caring" person in today's sense: the term would have meant nothing to him.' Bailey was clearly an ologist, not an ician.

A photograph captured Bailey's demonic gaze, as disturbing as Aleister Crowley's. He went mad after his only child, a son (also called Hamilton), was killed at the age of fifteen in a horrific railway accident. Bailey was locked up in a psychiatric hospital for three years and was about to undergo lobotomy when he was given a trial of lithium, then a new drug. Three months later, he had responded 'miraculously'.

Marston described the circumstances of Bailey's death: 'He retired to Fuengirola in the South of Spain, where he built a villa. Bailey then developed obstructing colonic cancer, a condition that he had fully described in many books. He consulted various doctors in Spain and Gibraltar but because of his eminence and contentious personality he was an impossibly demanding patient to treat. In February 1961 he died of the very complications he had spent his life explaining how to avoid.'

'Modern surgery is so much a matter of teamwork that the concept of the great surgeon is now almost obsolete,' wrote Marston. Many of the 'great men' I worked for would now be sacked or struck off. How the modern team, composed of easy-going 'caring' co-workers, would have appalled Bailey.

I was feeling too miserable with my cold to attend the grand round: 'Building a Community of Improvers'. One needed to be in the peak of health for such *rá méis*.*

⌢

I began the task of clearing out case notes on private patients accumulated over two decades; any over eight years old could, according to the data protection legislation, be shredded. I had no recollection of many of these patients. I saw them once, did some tests, and discharged them. The last letter generally began with: 'His/her investigations are very reassuring.' When people asked me what I did for a living, I would say I was in the reassurance business.

Some, however, I recalled vividly. A young woman with colitis who was moribund when she arrived in the 'rooms' in the consultants' clinic on the ministry grounds where I saw private patients. Somehow, I managed to admit her directly to the intensive care unit; she had her colon removed that evening, and survived.

A man with the most bizarre self-inflicted disease I had ever seen: a true case of Munchausen's syndrome. He regularly injected himself with a dilute solution of his own faeces, causing highly unusual skin abscesses. Richard Asher would have relished this case. The man bullied his local family doctor, who colluded with this deception, too afraid to tell us what he knew. This GP rather gave the game away, however – deliberately? –

---

* Irish; literally 'mad talk', means gibberish or drivel, but with a larding of contempt. The phrase does not have a direct English equivalent.

when he sent the man to the emergency department with a referral note stating that his patient 'most definitely *does not* have Munchausen's syndrome'.

A woman in whom I had missed an opportunity to diagnose a rare and potentially life-threatening condition; this disease later declared itself unambiguously. Miraculously, she survived my neglect and the late diagnosis. She lived on, however, to experience a series of debilitating illnesses and to become the main carer of a demented husband. 'Don't bore your colleagues with anecdotes about an imaginary golden age,' a distinguished older friend once advised me. 'Instead, tell them about your worst mistakes.'

'What do I do *now*?'

An emergency department consultant called, asking if I would give his trainees a tutorial on PEG tubes. His department had been phoned several times over the previous weekend by nursing homes asking for advice on these tubes, which were prone to block and leak.

'Don't you have someone who *deals* with this?' he asked incredulously.

'Most big hospitals would have a nutrition nurse to look after the PEG tubes, but we don't.'

'Why not?'

'I gave up asking for a nutrition nurse when the management decided to appoint a *latex allergy* nurse. I felt like Tom Lehrer.'

'Tom who?'

'Tom Lehrer gave up comedy when Henry Kissinger won the Nobel Peace Prize. He said the award had made political satire obsolete.'

I was still miserable with my cold, but the ward round was mercifully short. Some benign force, I thought, had taken 'pity on the least of things'. Little Tommy was back at the ministry; now that he had declined the transplant, I could promise that he would be home for Christmas. There was a knock on the door – a young man in a wheelchair; this was Mattie, a dialysis patient. He and Little Tommy had met at the smokers' huddle and become friends. Off they went, Little Tommy pushing Mattie, like figures from Beckett.

⌒

The ministry had an art collection, much of which consisted of acrylic portraits of doleful-looking farm animals and dramatic landscapes of the west Cork coast. Prominent in this collection was a large yellow abstract steel sculpture (*'Untitled'*) by the sculptor John Burke; this was placed at a roundabout near my office on the ministry grounds. When Burke died in 2006, *The Irish Times* reported: 'Known for his strongly individualistic nature, he asked to be buried in a standing position on a height in Co. Cork but within view of his native Co. Tipperary. Accordingly, he was buried in a standing position at Árd na Gaoithe cemetery, Watergrasshill, with a view of the Knock-mealdowns and the Galtee mountains.'

⌒

Strolling back to my office, I was stopped – no, *ambushed* – by a fellow consultant whose oleaginous and insincere conversation

I always tried to avoid. But there was no dodging her: no matter what route I took to my office, she would emerge from the corners and the shadows, with her vulpine, toothy rictus. A friend, whose loathing of this woman was all-consuming, once – only half-jokingly – suggested that she had been *cloned*, and four copies of her patrolled the ministry. It was almost plausible: when I occasionally went out the back entrance – as opposed to my usual route through the front – there she would be, asking whether I had been on holiday yet, and was the on-call very busy last night? She stalked the corridors at all hours, which prompted some speculation about her domestic circumstances.

Few things (the exceptions being titles and merit awards*) motivated British hospital doctors as much as the prospect of illicit sex. When I worked there, they were forever running

* Merit awards (now called 'Clinical Excellence Awards') were among the inducements given to hospital consultants by Aneurin Bevan to gain their support for the foundation of the NHS in 1948. 'I stuffed their mouths with gold,' he famously remarked. These awards 'reward the consultants who contribute most to the delivery of safe and high-quality care and the improvement of NHS services'. There are various levels of award; the highest ('platinum') effectively doubles the lucky recipient's salary. These awards were designed to reward those who did all the committee work, research, teaching and service development *on top of* their regular clinical activities; in reality, most of these awards are given to those who do this work *instead of* these unglamorous duties.

If there were merit awards in Ireland, Maurice would undoubtedly have a platinum award. Luckily – because the doctors would *kill* each other in pursuit of these baubles – we don't.

off with their secretaries, their nurses, their registrars, each other. It never seemed to make them any happier. Banished from the deep comfort of the marital home, they became estranged from their children and looked foolish.

I naively believed that this fever hadn't taken hold in Ireland until a friend put me right. Over a drink, he listed, with some relish, the names of our colleagues who had voluntarily left, or been thrown out of, the family home. Mostly men, mostly about fifty.

A famous musician was once admitted under my care with pneumonia. Years before, he had abandoned his first wife and many children for a young, beautiful woman. They married and moved into a small apartment. Not long after, he had a major stroke, which left him permanently disabled. When he recovered from this pneumonia, his wife asked me: 'What do I do *now*?' The lot of the second wife: hospital appointments, nursing homes.

The pianist

The first patient at the clinic was a man of eighty-five, referred to me by his GP, even though he lived five minutes' walk from his local hospital, seventy miles away. The poor man was agitated by this referral to a strange hospital and discommoded by the long bus journey. He had mentioned in passing to his GP that he very occasionally coughed and spluttered when he swallowed. She referred him to the speech and language therapists at the local hospital; they concluded that he had 'a severe problem at the upper oesophageal sphincter'. This alarming diagnosis was communicated to both patient and GP, who decided that he would need to be sent to the ministry. I did my best to reassure him that I did not think there was anything seriously amiss, but this message was difficult to convey through the fog of his deafness and agitation.

An email announced that today was European Antibiotic Awareness Day. The chief executive of the health service asked us 'to participate in stopping the spread of antibiotic-resistant superbugs through promoting smarter antibiotic use'. This chief executive was new; I wondered if he knew that only two months before, we'd had World Sepsis Day (marked by the illumination of the pyramids), urging us all to not hold back with the antibiotics? Whose guidance, I wanted to ask him, should we follow: his, or Dr Tedros Ghebreyesus, the director general of the WHO? Which cause was more worthy of my awareness: sepsis or antibiotic overuse?

My first patient on the ward round was a man in his eighties who regularly attended our clinic with chronic liver disease; he had come in with a chest infection. He was a pianist; he had delicate, beautiful hands. A small, frail man, he had gradually lost weight with the liver disease and old age. The dieticians were pressing my team to insert a nasogastric tube for feeding. I told them to resist this pressure; the man was dying.

The 'allied health professionals' – dieticians, physiotherapists, speech and language therapists, pharmacists – were becoming increasingly assertive with the junior doctors. I wearily reminded my team, almost daily, that these professionals would never be the ones to deal with the fallout, to have the difficult conversation or appear at an inquest; the only professional's name on the patient's sticker was *mine*.

I had coffee with two academics. One mentioned that the research output of a rival medical school had increased by 15 per cent, while ours had risen by only 3 per cent. He used the phrase 'research output' like a soviet commissar describing steel production. The ministry had taken on a distinctly Stalinist flavour over the previous few years, with its slogans, targets and five-year plans, its posters of Stakhanovite workers, the deliberate burial of bad news and disobliging facts, this pretence that we were all comrades, the cynical apparatchiks, the phoney worker participation, the *Pravda*-like newsletters, the Potemkin wards hastily cleared of patients on trolleys before external inspections. It stopped short, however, of a personality cult based around the chief executive.

The grand round was given by a young man from the business school of a Dublin university; his topic was digital health. He did that distracting TED Talk thing of pacing while he spoke; he paused – for theatrical effect – rather too frequently. I could only remember phrases, jargon: 'waterfall approach versus iterative approach'; 'data-rich but insight-poor and siloed'; 'informating'. A collaborator was described as a 'nursing informatician'; he referred to 'data' throughout his talk in the singular.

Andrea Pirlo's rich chestnut hair

World Pressure Ulcer Prevention Day. In the canteen, a wound nurse (who specialized in the treatment of patients with leg ulcers and pressure sores) encouraged me to enter a quiz on this topic.

〜♪

I was due to travel that weekend to Bellagio on Lake Como to attend a symposium on death; following the publication of my book *The Way We Die Now*, I was often invited to such gatherings. As I was packing, my phone rang; the medical registrar on call wanted to speak with me. She began with the once-dreaded phrase: 'I know you're not on call but ...' This phrase had been the overture to many episodes of unwelcome intrusion over the years; now I did not care. The pianist, as expected, had died. The registrar wanted to know if she should inform the coroner; any death even remotely connected with alcohol had to be reported. The pianist's liver disease might or might not have been alcohol-related; we weren't sure, because he never admitted that he drank heavily. Did it matter now? Would medicine, or society, benefit from the coroner's involvement? No, I said, the coroner doesn't need to know about the pianist. He's had quite enough, I thought, and so have I.

⟨ ⟩

On the flight from London to Milan, I saw Andrea Pirlo* sitting in the front row. I wasn't sure at first, but we made brief eye contact; yes, it was him. I told all the symposium participants about this sighting, but not one had heard of Andrea Pirlo. I could understand that people with no interest in football might not know of him, but two of our group had boasted of their allegiance to Wimbledon and Exeter City; surely, *they* should know who Andrea Pirlo was? Then again, to identify as a fan

---

* Andrea Pirlo (born 1979) won the World Cup with Italy in 2006; he played for several clubs, including Inter Milan, AC Milan and Juventus. Although Pirlo was slow and couldn't tackle, he made up for it with his composure, balance, technique and elegance. He had, in short, *sprezzatura*. Johan Cruyff called him 'a genius'. Because his game was not built on speed or physical strength, Pirlo continued playing at the very highest level into his late thirties.

During the COVID-19 lockdown of football, the *Guardian*'s football cartoonist David Squires produced a strip entitled 'Some random nice things about football'; one of these nice things was 'Andrea Pirlo's rich chestnut hair'. There has always been a homoerotic element in football fandom. I once met a man at a drinks party; we bonded over our admiration for Johan Cruyff. In 1974, when this man was a ten-year-old boy, he told his father that he loved Cruyff. 'Yes, he's a great player,' his father responded. 'No, no,' said the boy, 'you don't understand. I'm *in love* with Johan Cruyff.'

of clubs like these was to broadcast one's indifference – a *wilful and studied* indifference – to aristocrats like Pirlo.

News of Jonathan Miller's death; dementia took him, a cruel end. Despite his achievements, his fame, his reputation as the last 'polymath', he was not a happy man. He felt unfulfilled, bitterly regretting his failure to become the Nobel-Prize-winning neuroscientist he thought he should have been. 'I wasted my brilliant mind,' he once lamented. How dangerous early success can be: in his twenties, Miller had already been a member of the Cambridge 'Apostles' and a star of *Beyond the Fringe*. He had one last shot, in middle age, at medical research: studying perception, memory and cognition in brain-damaged people. It was a disaster: Miller lacked the patience, the doggedness, the capacity for enduring boredom and fail-ure that true science requires; he was too easily distracted. His published academic output from this sabbatical amounted to a single case report. Miller's problem was that he was a *fox* but wanted to be a *hedgehog*.* Why do people – particularly people as accomplished as Miller – want to be that which they are not?

Miller hated being called a 'polymath' or a 'renaissance man'; he thought these judgements were vulgar and glib. He was right. True polymaths are vanishingly rare; most

---

* This arbitrary bipartite division of mankind was propagated by Isaiah Berlin in *The Hedgehog and the Fox: An Essay on Tolstoy's View of History* (1953). He was inspired by a line from the Greek poet Archilochus: 'The fox knows many things, but the hedgehog knows one big thing.' Berlin wrote: 'Tolstoy was by nature a fox, but believed in being a hedgehog.' This 'systematic misinterpretation', he wrote, caused the novelist much pain: 'he is the most tragic of the great writers, a desperate old man, beyond human aid, wandering self-blinded at Colonus.'

so-called polymaths are mere dabblers. 'Polymath activities', wrote the biochemist and writer Carl Djerassi, 'must pass a certain level of quality control that is exerted within each field by the competition. If they accept you at their level, you have reached that stage rather than just dabbling.' A polymath must be the equal of the monomaths in each field of his or her activity. Miller was an opera director who happened to have a medical degree.

I spent five days at the Lucullan complex of gardens and villas in Bellagio; I met economists, philosophers, historians, film-makers, poets. Jonathan Miller would have loved it; how he would have lorded it at dinner.

I began to think of the world beyond, and the life after, the ministry of bodies.

⁓

The polymath test: Jonathan Miller failed, so too Oliver Sacks and Oliver St John Gogarty.* Neither Oliver was much respected by the monomaths within medicine: Sacks fled from mainstream academic neurology and published little in the specialist journals; Gogarty was a fashionable but mediocre ear, nose and throat surgeon whose contribution to the scientific literature (a single case report in the *British Medical Journal* in 1914[†]) was even slighter than Sacks's.

* Oliver St John Gogarty (1878–1957) was an Irish surgeon, poet, athlete, politician and wit. His lyric poems were much admired by W. B. Yeats. He is probably most famous for being the model for 'Buck Mulligan' in James Joyce's *Ulysses*.

† 'Latent empyema of the nasal accessory sinuses.'

*

Wilfred Trotter (1872–1939) is my idea of a medical polymath – in his own words, one of 'the small and sporadic crop of the heroically gifted'. Wilfred *who*? Trotter was, by common consent, the finest British surgeon of the interwar years. In 1928, he operated on George V for empyema (an abscess between the ribs and the lung), saving his life; he carried out the operation in Buckingham Palace, travelling there by bus. For this service, he was offered a knighthood, which he – rather stylishly – refused. Trotter was a pioneer in several branches of surgery, including neurosurgery and head and neck surgery. His contemporaries and students at University College Hospital (UCH) London regarded him with awe: 'no gentler hands were ever given to a surgeon,' wrote his pupil, the neurosurgeon Julian Taylor. Robin Pilcher, one of his protégés, described him as 'the perfect example of a good doctor'.

Trotter's *Instincts of the Herd in Peace and War* (1915) was a major contribution to social psychology. The book coined the phrase 'the herd instinct' and influenced many, including Edward Bernays (Sigmund Freud's nephew, a pioneer of propaganda, public relations and advertising). He was one of the first in Britain to recognise the importance of Freud, although he later criticised him for ignoring the social aspects of psychology. When Freud was dying of cancer in London, Trotter was asked to see him.

He was a prose stylist: 'He used the English language as he used his hands,' said a colleague, 'with a delicate precision born of constant striving after perfect control.' Although Trotter is most remembered for *Instincts of the Herd*, his later essays (*Collected Papers*), on what might broadly be called the philosophy of science, are better. He was both aloof and charismatic; his approach to teaching and conversation was Socratic, questioning received opinion: 'The mind likes a strange idea as little as the body likes a strange protein, and resists it with similar energy.' Addressing a class of students commencing their training at UCH in 1932, Trotter told them to think for themselves (an unusual exhortation to medical students): 'Uniformity of thought is an increasingly apparent goal and demand of civilization. Still there burns on in most of us a small wild spark. I advise you to nourish it as a precious possession. Really to think for oneself is as strange, difficult and dangerous as any adventure.'

Trotter was, I think, a hunchback. As a teenager, he contracted spinal 'caries' (tuberculosis), spending years confined to bed. He recovered, but, according to the physician Douglas Holdstock, 'had a perpetual stoop, making him appear well below average height'.

Raymond Tallis (born 1946) is probably the only polymath lurking in contemporary medicine: professor of geriatrics, philosopher, public intellectual, not to mention Kirsty Young's favourite castaway on *Desert Island Discs*. Described as the most respected philosopher never to have held an academic position in the subject, he did this work every day between 5 and 7 a.m., before setting off to start his day as a doctor. To be a polymath, you need to be not only 'heroically gifted' but also an early riser.

The word *sprezzatura* first appeared in Baldassare Castiglione's *The Book of the Courtier* (1528); he defined it as 'a certain non-chalance, so as to conceal all art and make whatever one does or says appear to be without effort and almost without any thought about it'.

Reviewing his friend Oliver Sacks's memoir *On the Move*, the neurologist Andrew Lees wrote: 'Aspirant British neurologists of his generation were often reminded by their chiefs to be never seen running on duty. They were expected to be effete, clubbable, cerebral and graceful.'

I dreamed about Jonathan Miller. I took him to a bookshop, where I bought him a copy of my book *Can Medicine Be Cured?*

'*That's* what "abnormal" means'

Far from Andrea Pirlo and the gardens of Bellagio, I started the outpatient clinic with Declan, the man with long-standing 'medically unexplained symptoms'. When I last saw him, his main concern was food intolerance; he was now requesting that he be tested for 'toxins', which he believed were contaminating his food. Although he was now forty and not intellectually disabled, his mother always accompanied him to the clinic, but remained in the waiting room. He had resisted when I last saw him, but Declan now gave his cautious, conditional assent to a referral to liaison psychiatry.

Next in was The Angriest Man in Ireland, who had suffered with irritable bowel syndrome for thirty-five years. He told me that he was now housebound, that his life was not worth living. Despite this, he had travelled, within the previous year, to India, Canada and Australia. He emptied onto the desk, rather insolently, a bag containing his medications; there were fifteen boxes. I told him I did not wish to add to this pile.

'I'm sorry I can't help more,' I said wearily. To my astonishment, The Angriest Man in Ireland *also* agreed to a referral to liaison psychiatry.

I reviewed Marie with chronic abdominal pain, the woman who had summoned a medium to her house. The spirits summoned by this medium, you will recall, had very obligingly told Marie that this pain would eventually dissipate, but somehow it had persisted, in defiance of the reassurances given by her dead relatives. Marie's GP had finally nudged her towards acceptance of a psychological origin of her pain. She showed me the sheet of paper on which her GP had drawn the components making up the vicious circle driving her pain. I could make out the phrase 'disturbs quality of life'. Marie, too, agreed to a psychiatry referral.

I paused to reflect on how I had referred three of my most refractory patients to psychiatry. This was not remarkable; what was remarkable was that they had all *agreed*.

In the afternoon, a woman attended for colonoscopy; she had no friends or relatives, so had the procedure without sedation, and planned to get the bus home. Her colonoscopy was normal.

'What do you mean it's *normal*?' she asked tetchily.

'I mean I didn't find any abnormality. I didn't find any disease,' I said brightly. 'That's generally good news.'

'So why am I constipated?'

*

A man, whom I confidently reassured at clinic that his bleeding was probably due to haemorrhoids, had a large cancer of the rectum. How I wished I could tell the last woman: 'See? *That's* what "abnormal" means.'

A cold grey day, a long slow ward round. My first patient was an elderly demented woman with pneumonia and respiratory failure; her face was obscured by the BiPAP* mask. Her son questioned me closely. There had been some disagreement about resuscitation the week before between one of my colleagues and the family. I avoided the issue.

'Have you decided yet what to do with me?' asked a grand, well-spoken old man. He had a muscular spasm on the left side of his face, which gave the unfortunate and unintended impression of winking. I noticed he was reading *The Spectator*; this was the first time I had ever seen a patient reading this magazine. Patients' reading material was often a good guide to their cognitive abilities, as well as an excuse to talk to them about their lives. I had often learned a great deal by asking: 'What's that you're reading?'

* Bilevel Positive Airway Pressure, a form of non-invasive ventilation that delivers oxygen under pressure.

*

Pat, a man with alcoholic liver disease, was dying in what the nurses called the 'death bed' (first on the left in the ward's observation unit). He was only fifty-seven but looked much older. Earlier in the day, he became acutely distressed with breathlessness, but this settled with morphine. His sister and brother-in-law were at his bedside, with a tray of tea and biscuits. I had spoken with this sister on several occasions, trying to nudge her towards an acceptance that Pat was going to die, but she found it difficult to grasp what I was telling her. After our last conversation, she came back to the ward and told the team that she was happy for me to make all the decisions.

The gynaecologist said she was 'too busy' to come to the ward through the link corridor from her base in the maternity hospital to see my patient with vaginal bleeding; she relayed this message via her specialist nurse. Instead, she would conduct a *telephone consultation* with the patient. I wondered how she would carry out a pelvic examination.

'There's nothing like a difficult patient to show us ourselves'

The general medical 'take' was small, only seven patients. I struggled to conceal my irritation with the senior house officer who ate a banana while she presented the first case, her mouth stuffed with food as she spoke. This was a man with a complicated hip problem, for which he was attending the orthopaedic service. He had come in, he said, because the pain was now unbearable. The orthopaedic surgeon on call, who had done his rounds even earlier than me, refused to take him. I phoned another consultant, the man's regular orthopaedic surgeon; he agreed to take him, but called me back an hour later to say that if he'd known that the on-call surgeon had refused to take the patient, *he* would have refused too. A year before, I might have reacted to such provocation; now, I couldn't care less. I reflected, with some regret, on the countless episodes of such petty professional turf wars I had been involved in over my years at the ministry. Each one had chipped away a little of my regard for my fellow doctors.

*

Pat, the man with alcoholic liver disease in the 'death bed', died, as expected, overnight; his bed was quickly filled by Michael, another man with the same disease. He was from Birmingham and moved to Cork in the mid-1990s to marry an Irishwoman; she had died a couple of years before. Two of his brothers had died of alcohol-related diseases. After his wife's death, Michael continued the family tradition and took to drink, consuming two three-litre flagons of cider a day; his flat was conveniently located next door to a supermarket. He was now deeply jaundiced and his kidneys were failing. His only relative was a dull stepson.

'I'm going to get better,' Michael said. 'I'm going to *fight* it.'

I came across an article on 'difficult' patients and 'difficult' encounters; the authors of this essay estimated that fifteen per cent of clinical encounters are 'difficult'. I wondered how many thousands of such episodes I had experienced over thirty-six years. 'There's nothing like a difficult patient', wrote William Carlos Williams, 'to show us ourselves.'

Williams (1883–1963) was an American poet and physician. He worked as a family doctor for four decades in a poor neighbourhood of Rutherford, New Jersey. He published many collections of modernist poetry, as well as novels, short stories, art criticism, history, and an autobiography. He was posthumously awarded the Pulitzer Prize for his 1962 collection *Pictures from Brueghel*.

In his *Autobiography* (1951), Williams wrote: 'As a writer I have never felt that medicine interfered with me but rather that it was my very food and drink, the very thing which made it possible for me to write.' This is a common, comforting narrative of doctor-writers. His son, William Eric Williams, in his essay 'My Father, the Doctor', told a different, heartbreaking story, of 'a man making his living at medicine who has given up medicine for poetry' and who called his medical work 'a hellish drag'.

Williams's tragedy was that old problem – *sustenance*. Williams's friend Ezra Pound urged him to abandon medicine and move to Europe. He spent some time in Vienna after the First World War, and later, in the early 1920s, visited France. By then, he had a young family, and decided that poverty was not for him; the pram was already in the hall. He would never, he concluded, make an adequate living from writing alone.

Williams had a horror of bohemia. It was more than the unwashed dishes piled up in the sink or the unpaid bills: 'What I could never tolerate in Pound or seek for myself was the "side" that went with all his posturings as the poet. To me that was the emptiest of old hat.' Williams's medical training, his 'upbringing', he wrote, gave him 'the humility and caution of the scientist'.

Williams must have been a man of boundless energy, because in addition to his writing and doctoring, he had an extraordinarily busy sex life. 'I am extremely sexual in my desires,' he wrote in *Autobiography*; 'I carry them everywhere and at all times.' He recalled how, as a medical student, he had fallen in love with the corpse of a beautiful mixed-race woman, 'lying stripped on the dissecting table before me'. T. S. Eliot would have fainted at the prospect.

Did William Carlos Williams have sexual relationships with his *patients?* Bethel Solomons (1885–1965) was an eminent Irish gynaecologist, who observed in his memoir *One Doctor in His Time* (1956) that 'women definitely prefer to have handsome men around them when they are having babies'. (Judging by the surviving photographs of him, Solomons was a strikingly good-looking man.) This kind of attention, however, could be risky: 'I always warn young doctors, particularly if they are good-looking, that they cannot be too careful to maintain decorum in their relations with women patients. Women ask the most extraordinary things. On two occasions, at least, I have been asked by women patients, whose husbands were sterile, to oblige them. Needless to say, I refused these open invitations, in the same way as I have refused several insinuated ones.' Did Solomons, I wonder, give this advice to 'good-looking' young doctors only, or did he proffer it also – so as not to hurt their feelings – to his more homely trainees?

William Carlos Williams and Jonathan Miller shared a belief that art should celebrate the everyday, the overlooked, the un-glamorous. Miller called it 'finding the considerable in the negligible'. Williams wrote that this art was far from easy: 'the thing that stands eternally in the way of really good writing is always one: the virtual impossibility of lifting to the imagination those things which lie under the direct scrutiny of the senses, close to the nose. It is this difficulty that sets a value upon all works of art and makes them a necessity.'

All I want for Christmas

An old man I had seen on several occasions over the years walked into my consulting room in the clinic wearing tracksuit bottoms, pushing a tri-wheel mobility aid; he acquired this following a fall the year before. He was now bothered with constipation and was very anxious to have this investigated; I agreed to book him for a colonoscopy. He had no one to collect him, he said, could I bring him in for a couple of nights? I told him that this would be difficult to arrange, that he might have to wait three months or more for his colonoscopy. I could feel my irritation mounting, but then evaporate, and turn to pity; this lonely old man did not have a child or a friend to carry out this simple service for him.

A man was referred with loss of appetite and weight loss. I examined his abdomen; there was an enormous craggy mass filling most of his belly. This was his liver, stuffed with cancerous deposits. His GP had not bothered to examine him before referring.

Anticipating a large attendance, the Schwartz round was held in the main lecture theatre; the theme was 'Christmas'. The facilitator asked us *not* to applaud the speakers. The first was a geriatrics registrar, who told a rather pointless story about a frail old man called 'Patrick'. He was admitted to hospital, discharged to a nursing home, where he died three months later. 'Nobody asked Patrick what was important to him,' she said mournfully.

A surgeon, who seemed embarrassed to be taking part, talked about a young man who, before he died, gave him the gift of a watch, 'to thank you for your time'. To everyone's surprise, he hesitated, briefly losing his usual composure, his voice catching with emotion.

Last, a nurse who had taken orphaned children on holiday. On the flight, two little boys pointed at the clouds, asking if their mammies were in heaven, and did they know each other? Both mammies had died of heroin addiction.

'Would anyone like to share a memory of Christmas?' the facilitator asked hopefully. A long uncomfortable silence was broken by a nurse who spoke about setting up a 'hugging rota' for a man dying of leukaemia. 'We set up a WhatsApp group,' she explained.

I wondered what I would say if the facilitator asked *me* to share a memory. Christmas had no 'special' memories for me. I had worked many Christmas Days. I did not especially resent this; what I hated was that the period over Christmas and the New Year was like a weekend on call, but a weekend that went on for *two weeks*. Every Christmas Day, I thought of Patricia, the young woman who had died of liver failure on that day in 2001. Every New Year's Eve, I thought of the doctor who died of an aortic dissection, diagnosed too late. I was not tempted to share these memories.

Is there anything more useless than good intentions?

Michael – the man with alcoholic liver disease in the 'death bed' – was slowly dying. He was deeply jaundiced, and his kidneys were failing. I had decided early on not to send Michael to the intensive care unit or for kidney dialysis. His only relative was his stepson, Jerry, who could not understand what I was telling him but was content for me to make the decisions.

'Thank you for your expertise, Professor'

Somerset Maugham was brave where William Carlos Williams hesitated. He qualified as a doctor, but never practised. In old age, he wrote: 'I think I learned pretty well everything I know about human nature in the 5 years I spent at St Thomas' Hospital.' Maugham endured a hard decade before any success as a writer. He later regretted this decision: 'I am sorry I abandoned medicine so soon. It was idiotic. Absolutely idiotic. I could as well have written at night and avoided the desperate financial struggle I had. I should have got the usual hospital appointments, gone as assistant to general practitioners in various parts of the country, and done locums; I should thus have acquired a mass of valuable experience.' It's difficult to imagine the fastidious and worldly Maugham working as a locum GP in some provincial town, writing in the evenings. He was only nine years older than Williams; while the younger man was slowly killing himself in Rutherford, New Jersey, Maugham surveyed the world he didn't much care for through those hooded reptilian eyes, from the comfort of the Villa Mauresque in Cap Ferrat. A weekend accompanying Williams on his house calls would have cured him of his regret about leaving medicine.

Maugham must confound the modern purveyors of empathy in medicine, with his unpredictable mixture of misanthropy and curiosity. 'Though I have never much liked men,' he wrote in *The Summing Up*, 'I have found them so interesting that I am almost incapable of being bored by them.' He accepted with equanimity his position in 'the top rank of the second rate', concluding that it was his punishment for *entertaining* his vast readership: 'There can be nothing so gratifying to an author as to arouse the respect and esteem of the reader. Make him laugh and he will think you a trivial fellow, but bore him in just the right way and your reputation is assured.'

Somerset Maugham and Wilfred Trotter studied medicine at different London hospitals around the same time. Maugham was at St Thomas' from 1892 to 1897; Trotter was at UCH from 1891 to 1896. I don't think they ever met, but I like to think they would have hit it off. Like Maugham, Trotter didn't much care for people, but he was fascinated by them. 'The peculiar quality of his approach to the sick,' wrote Julian Taylor, 'was a gentleness that had nothing of the feminine, nor roots in affection for his fellows.' Like Maugham, Trotter was 'almost pathologically reserved'; like Maugham, he was renowned for his 'outrageously well-aimed and piercing witticisms'. As writers, they share an appealing, vinegary quality.

It was my last ever weekend night on call. I was not surprised, as I was eating dinner, when the hospital switchboard phoned and put through the medical registrar. A liver patient was deteriorating; she was worried.

'Would you like me to come in?'

'Well, I *am* worried.'

The patient was a woman of about sixty, skinny and tattooed, with alcoholic cirrhosis, admitted with a severe pneumonia. Since Michael had died overnight, *she* now occupied the 'death bed'. She was drowsy, having been given a sedative injection before a CT scan of her chest and abdomen. The medical registrar was under the impression that she was on the 'active' liver transplant list, meaning that she might be summoned at any moment to the liver unit in Dublin. I thought this unlikely; a call to one of the liver unit consultants confirmed that she was not. I took her husband aside to tell him that we were doing everything we could, but she might not survive.

As I left the ward, a Filipina nurse who had worked on the ward for many years put her hand on my shoulder, smiled and said: 'Thank you for your expertise, Professor.' I felt strangely moved, as if she were thanking me for a lifetime's work.

On the drive home, I recalled how this nurse – one of the most gentle people I had ever known – was once verbally abused by a grieving relative at a meeting convened by the ministry's risk management department after this relative complained about her late mother's care. I watched the tears roll down the nurse's face – for this was a great injustice – and silently cursed the ministry (and myself) for not supporting her. It was an unwritten rule at the ministry that bereaved relatives could say *anything* without being challenged.

I reached the emergency department the next morning before 7.00; it was crowded and chaotic. My first patient was an elderly man on a trolley by the nurses' station. He turned when I approached. 'Is that *you*, Seamus?' He had been my teacher decades ago; how diminished he looked now. Back then, he had a demonic thwarted energy; this energy often found an outlet in violence. On one occasion, I was subjected to a beating, having been caught talking to another boy while he was out of the classroom taking a phone call. He ordered me to bend over, took a short run up, and kicked my buttocks so hard that I briefly became airborne. I had forgotten this painful event until many years later when I watched the famous 'Kicking Bishop Brennan Up the Arse' episode in *Father Ted*. The trauma counsellors will be disappointed to learn that I bore the teacher little ill will; all I felt now was pity.

The Christmas display on the main corridor featured the usual animals (the cattle, a donkey, some sheep) reputed to have been in the stable in Bethlehem. Included also in this tableau was a proud-looking penguin, several fawns, a polar bear cub perched on the back of an adult bear, and yet another polar bear, climbing – rather improbably – up a Christmas tree.

Diogenes

I received a letter about Felix from a liaison psychiatrist, the same psychiatrist whose lecture on the management of patients with medically unexplained symptoms I had attended a couple of years before: 'Felix believes that he is suffering from a medical condition that the doctors are aware of but have not disclosed to him. He made it clear that he would not come back to the clinic as he does not believe that he has any mental health problems.'

I rather admired Felix's consistency; did his obstinate resistance cause the psychiatrist to rethink her facile ideas about the management of patients with 'medically unexplained symptoms'?

⌒

A young man – a junior manager – at the entrance to the canteen gave me a sheet detailing 'The five fundamentals of unscheduled care'. 'Unscheduled' was now the word preferred by the managerial classes to 'acute' or 'emergency'. I asked him if this document contained any mention of extra beds. 'It's about *process*,' he said, 'not *structure*.'

I lunched with a surgeon. He told me about a patient, a Jehovah's Witness, who needed a major operation. He came to the clinic with his wife and an 'advisor' from his church. The patient asked to see the surgeon alone. He told him: 'If I need blood, give it, but don't tell them. I'd be ostracised if they found out.'

The first patient on the ward round was an old lady in a single room on my home ward. She had come in with jaundice, which was caused by a pancreatic cancer obstructing her bile duct. We had decompressed this bile duct blockage by inserting a stent endoscopically, and her jaundice was settling. Her daughter bore a perpetual appearance of worry and dread. 'She was very vague and listless today,' she told me. 'What could be causing that?' I paused; I was tempted to reply: 'She's ninety-three. She has dementia. She has pancreatic cancer.' But I didn't. Instead, I give her platitudinous stuff about taking things slowly, one day at a time.

I went to the intensive care unit to see a man who had been admitted with a severe pneumonia and kidney failure. He lived alone in squalor. He had fallen in his small flat and was on the ground for many hours. He eventually managed to phone 999 and got through to the police, who broke down the door. On the way to hospital, he had a cardiac arrest, and was miraculously resuscitated. I mentioned to the team that this man might be given a label of Diogenes syndrome* – a combination of self-neglect, social isolation, squalor and obsessive hoarding ('syllogomania').

'There were two philosophers called Diogenes,' said Stanislaus, my Polish senior house officer. 'I think this one was Diogenes the Cynic.'

'How did you know that?' I asked.

---

* The syndrome is badly named, for the Greek philosopher Diogenes (d. 323 BC) was not 'socially isolated' – he was an enthusiastic public masturbator – and he was not a hoarder, his only possession being a barrel or, possibly, a clay wine jar. The geriatricians now prefer the term 'senile squalor syndrome'. The eponymous naming of diseases and syndromes is now frowned upon; there will never be a new condition named 'O'Mahony's syndrome'.

The poet Nicholas Moore (son of the philosopher G. E.), who died in 1986, fulfilled all the criteria for Diogenes syndrome, and raised failure to the level of an art form. The literary academic Peter Howarth wrote an appreciation for the *London Review of Books* in 2015: 'Moore's last years were spent in a purposeful shambles. The poet Peter Riley visited him in 1984, and his account memorably describes the mounds of rubbish, food, records and paper that covered every available surface in the tiny flat. Some of these papers were Moore's own poems, which he would work at every day, all day, and then lose in the tottering piles or under the kitchen sink. Moore would ensure his continued non-success by sending in reams of doggerel to editors, in which might be concealed a few bits of perfectly struck poetry.'

W. H. Auden's domestic arrangements were almost as shambolic. He believed that this way of living was necessary for his art: 'I hate living in squalor – I detest it! – but I can't do the work I want to do and live any other way.' Stravinsky said of Auden: 'He is the dirtiest man I have ever liked.'

'In Poland, classical history and philosophy are taught in the schools.'

Stanislaus was a man of many, sometimes unexpected, accomplishments. He was often the interpreter for his compatriots; he could also speak serviceable Russian.

My last case of Diogenes syndrome was an elderly man who, on a Saturday afternoon, had been bundled into an ambulance at the insistence of his relatives and neighbours, and deposited on a trolley in the emergency department. As I was on 'take' for the weekend, he became my 'patient'. I asked him who his nearest relative was.

'My cat.'

'What's your cat's name?'

'She has no fucking name.'

A trystorm

I attended a lunchtime training session in the main lecture theatre on 'the five fundamentals of unscheduled care'. The event was introduced by the new chief executive, who handed over to Rita from the special delivery unit at the Dublin head-quarters of the Irish Health Service Executive. Rita cheerfully admitted that all her ideas had been nicked from NHS Scot-land. 'More than process,' she beamed, 'it's about winning hearts and minds. Data and business intelligence are core.' Rita concluded with the new folksy, Pollyannaish mantra of health service managers: 'It's better to light a candle than curse the darkness.' She handed over to Simon from a management consultancy firm, who proclaimed they could 'deliver solu-tions to all business challenges'. Simon passed the baton on to Teddy, a psychiatric nurse who had risen without trace to become a senior manager; his almost comic inarticulacy had not hindered this ascent.

A geriatrician – stethoscope draped around his neck, as if he had rushed here from the emergency department – showed us a Heath Robinson slide entitled 'The Ambulatory

Care Pathway', which had been 'thrashed out' after two weeks of meeting with 'all stakeholders'. He talked for some considerable time, deploying phrases such as 'enhanced front door team', 'older person co-ordinator' and 'rapid ambulatory assessment clinic'. Slyly and stealthily, he inched his way to the revelation that the solution to the trolley crisis – a crisis that had dogged Irish health care for two decades now – was *more geriatricians*: 'frail old people need to come under the right team'.

A short study, conducted over three days, was proof enough. The geriatrician had organised a trystorm,* a three-day experiment during which the emergency department was flooded with geriatricians, 'frailty nurse specialists', occupational therapists and physiotherapists. 'We avoided twenty-one admissions,' he proudly declared. This astonishing result persuaded the new chief executive to fund the expansion of the geriatric service by one consultant, one registrar and a frailty nurse specialist. 'We need a proper frailty unit,' the geriatrician piously concluded. Given the enthusiasm with which the chief executive, Rita, Simon and Teddy clapped this conclusion, I predicted that such a unit would open very soon.

The speciality of geriatrics was developed in the 1960s and '70s by a few saintly pioneers, such as Marjory Warren and Bernard Isaacs. Many of the second wave of NHS geriatricians, however,

---

* A trystorm is 'a combination of brain-storming melded with rapid prototyping to determine if ideas will work quickly or not'.

were cynical and disillusioned; they did not subscribe to the speciality's quasi-religious belief that old age, frailty and death could be ameliorated, contained. One confessed to me that his main function was to make 'ethical' decisions. Many of them escaped and became clinical directors; some I knew rose to the most senior positions in the sharp-elbowed world of NHS management. No other speciality was so well represented in this milieu.

An elderly acquaintance of mine believed with the conviction of religious faith that age was, as the cliché would have it, 'a state of mind': the old only got old through *carelessness*.

My secretary left a message about a patient. A woman I had arranged to be admitted for investigation cancelled because she did not want to leave her dog. When I saw this woman at the outpatients, I strongly suspected she had a cancer. I phoned her GP. 'Dr Jim isn't in,' the receptionist said, 'but you can speak to his daughter.' We had an amiable conversation about how difficult this woman was.

All over the city and county, dutiful medical graduates were apprenticed to their parents, as if doctoring was a hereditary priesthood.

I gave an ethics tutorial to the final-year students; my theme was resuscitation. Afterwards, a student approached me.

'You seem like a very wise man,' he said. 'Can I ask you a question?'

'Sure,' I said, thinking that no one had ever called me 'wise'.

'How can I be sure if I'm being true to myself?'

I received an email from an old friend, a colleague from my NHS days. We were once close enough for him to ask me to be a groomsman at his wedding. He was now a prominent academic; I hadn't heard from him in years. I thought of Julian Barnes's bipartite division of people – a far better one than Isaiah Berlin's hedgehogs and foxes – into *narrativists* and *episodicists*. Narrativists believe that life is a story, with an arc and a meaning; episodicists (like me) see no unifying theme or meaning; stuff happens, then more stuff. People – like this friend – come and, very often, go. For the episodicist, the defining characteristic of human life is absurdity.

I first met this friend in Bradford. We worked for a physician who liked to play the role of professional Yorkshireman. I once heard this exchange between him and a ward sister at St Luke's Hospital:

Ward sister: 'Where are ya goin' on yer 'olidays, doctor?'
Doctor: 'To Blackpool, to see illuminations.'

An interview panel was convened to appoint senior house officers for the ministry's internal medicine training scheme. One candidate divided the panel. The chairwoman remarked, in an entirely neutral, curious manner, that the panel was split along gender lines. 'Women see things more *holistically*,' said a woman panellist.

'My visits here are largely ceremonial'

'You're too young to retire,' said the first man at the out-patients, generously. 'I liked you; you had a gentle way.'

A Polish woman pulled up her T-shirt and pointed at her belly: 'Like a balloon, like a ball!' Like many of her compatriots, she had travelled home to Poland to have an endoscopy. I asked her how much this cost: 'Seventeen euro. Thirty if you have anaesthetic.'

The Polish endoscopist had taken some biopsies from her stomach and duodenum; she showed me the report. I could just about make out – Polish medical terminology is Latin-based – that the duodenal biopsy showed a slight elevation in the population of intraepithelial lymphocytes. This can be a subtle manifestation of coeliac disease, caused by gluten sensitivity. This mild abnormality is sometimes called 'Marsh I' after the gastroenterologist* who described it. The report referred to '*Marsha* I'.

'You know what is *Marsha*?'

'I knew Marsh well,' I was tempted to say, 'and wasted the best years of my life counting intraepithelial lymphocytes.' But I did not; I just confirmed that yes, I knew what 'Marsha' was, and asked her what the Polish doctors advised her to do.

'I go before result,' she shrugged. 'I was on holiday.'

A Chinese man was referred with dyspepsia. Although he had lived in Ireland for thirty years, his daughter had to interpret for him. Since his GP had referred him, he too had gone to his homeland for tests – to Hong Kong, where he'd had a gastroscopy. He showed me the report – complete with several Polaroids of his stomach – which gave a dramatic combined diagnosis of 'severe oesophagitis, gastritis and duodenitis'. His oesophagus, stomach and duodenum looked pristinely healthy on the Polaroids. The doctors in Hong Kong clearly believed that *paying* patients did not want to be told that everything was 'normal'.

⌣⁓

---

* Michael Marsh, formerly reader in gastroenterology at Hope Hospital, Salford. He classified the severity of the small intestinal mucosal abnormality in coeliac disease. There are four stages in this classification, ranging from 'Marsh I' (the mildest) to 'Marsh IV' (the most severe). In retirement, Marsh worked at Oxford University on the theology and neurophysiology of near-death and out-of-body experiences.

I did my ward round in the afternoon. The team told me that the family of an elderly woman who had been on the ward for over six weeks was vehemently opposed to any suggestion of a DNACPR (do not attempt cardio-pulmonary resuscitation) order. I examined her while her son stood anxiously by the bedside. I funked the inevitable, quite necessary, confrontation, reasoning that because she was gradually improving, this difficult conversation could wait. 'We'll deal with that when we have to,' I said, convincing no one, including myself.

A man who had been in for several weeks complained of back pain; an MRI scan showed discitis – infection in one of the intervertebral discs. A specialist in infectious diseases had seen him; he wrote a long note, but without giving any clear recommendation. I phoned Con, my microbiologist friend, who told me that I should get a radiologist to take a sample from the infected disc for culture (to isolate the bacterium causing the infection), and that I should do this quickly. I persuaded a neuroradiologist to do it later that morning.

All this, I fumed, should have been done the day before, or even the day before that, when the MRI result was available, but the registrar had been dragged off to help at a clinic, and then went home sick, leaving only the intern to cover the wards. I would soon be leaving, I thought; I no longer had the stomach to make an issue of it.

A man with lung cancer had a huge fluid collection in his right lung. He was now short of breath even at rest; he needed the urgent insertion of a chest drain.

'We can't do that today,' said my registrar, 'he's on warfarin. He might bleed if we put in a chest drain.'

'Why is he on warfarin?'

'Atrial fibrillation.'*

This man was on warfarin to reduce the risk of a stroke in his non-existent future. Dying people, I had noticed, often continued to consume 'preventive' medications such as anti-coagulants, statins, aspirin and drugs for high blood pressure. Did their doctors continue these drugs to avoid difficult conversations?

Diogenes in the intensive care unit, the recluse who had been rescued by the police, was slightly better, but his survival would be a pyrrhic victory. If he lived, he would be left in a persistent vegetative state, his brain having been deprived of oxygen for several minutes while he was resuscitated in the ambulance on the way to hospital. The intensive care duty consultant asked if I had anything to add. 'No,' I said. 'My visits here are largely ceremonial.'

---

* Atrial fibrillation is a common disorder of heart rhythm that can cause a stroke by forming a blood clot within one of the chambers of the heart, which can then travel (embolise) to the brain. Anticoagulants (blood thinners) such as warfarin are commonly prescribed to reduce this risk.

A good death

A large group of young Travellers gathered at the front entrance of the ministry. Their conversation was conducted at maximum volume, everyone shouting. How solicitous they were for their sick, how warm their communality. They breezily ignored the booming recorded voice that admonished them for smoking in the vicinity of the breast unit.

⁓

The shopping centre on the opposite side of the main road to the ministry had not changed since the 1980s: low, oppressive ceilings, cheap shops, tatty cafés. The day was mild, damp and overcast, which added to a gloom that was indifferent to the proximity of Christmas. A woman wearing a tiny Santa hat, perched on her head at an angle, approached me in Tesco. 'You probably don't remember me,' she said, 'but I'm one of your fifty thousand patients.' I *did* recognise her; it was the Santa hat.

A letter came from the hospice, informing me of the death of one of my patients, a woman with oesophageal cancer. The palliative care registrar wrote: 'She was initially restless and agitated secondary to significant spiritual distress. However, she was unable to engage with pastoral care as she was too fatigued. After discussion with her family, she was commenced on a continuous subcutaneous infusion for management of these symptoms.' It was wonderful how mortal terror – 'spiritual distress' – could be magicked away by morphine and midazolam delivered by 'continuous subcutaneous infusion'. Medicine has yet to come up with a more useful drug than morphine; without it, few would have the heart to practise the profession.

I could not help feeling that this hospice doctor found my patient *wanting* in her failure to 'engage with pastoral care', that her dying merited only a C-minus. All this pressure, now, to have a 'good death'. I kept hearing the phrase 'successful dying'; I couldn't quite articulate why it irritated me so much. I think it was the implicit assumption on the part of these well-meaning professionals that they could tame the unknowable with their tick-box criteria, their workshops, their systematic reviews. No rage, please, *engage* with pastoral care.

A 2016 article published in an American geriatrics journal entitled 'Defining a Good Death (Successful Dying)' listed eleven 'core themes' of a good death, one of which was a miscellaneous 'other' category, which included 'having pets nearby'. According to these criteria, my father had a *bad death*: 'dying' in the resus room of an emergency department, after the futile attentions of the cardiac arrest team. I'm not so sure. He was dead by the time the ambulance arrived at our street, where he had collapsed. What happened subsequently when his body was subjected to this medical ritual cannot have caused *him* any suffering.

He was seventy-one when he died. He married late – at forty-six – twenty years older than my mother. He had his first heart attack in his mid-fifties, an event he tried to conceal. He had a second infarction in his late sixties. He refused to attend hospital on both occasions, but did consent to see an old-fashioned general physician, whose hands-off, minimally interventional approach suited him. For the last year of his life, he woke frequently at night with breathlessness due to heart failure – so-called paroxysmal nocturnal dyspnoea. I tried to persuade him to see a heart specialist, but he wouldn't hear of it. He hated fussing, he hated doctors, he hated hospitals, he hated illness. He would not have regarded his death as entirely unsatisfactory. Although he never articulated this fear, he dreaded the prospect of a prolonged illness, hospitalisation, and loss of independence. Like Ivan Illich (whom he had never heard of), he believed in the right to die without a diagnosis. He would have been appalled by the prospect of deathbed farewells: he regarded all displays of emotion as vulgar and unmanly. He would not have been keen on the inevitable visit of the priest for the last confession and the anointing with oil. He might have been amused that the cardiac arrest team in those days included the Catholic chaplain. By the time my father got to the resus room, he was gone. He died instantly on the street where he lived, while walking his dog. (At least he ticked one box in the good death criteria: 'proximity to pets'.) His death was traumatic for the rest of us, but not for him.

⌒

Brendan Behan: 'Death always has dignity. Maybe *dying* hasn't much dignity, but once dead, a man becomes defiant. You can no longer frighten him.'

⌒

We long for dignity and meaning, but the world gives us absurdity. Whenever a patient of mine died, something unseemly often happened: an inappropriate remark or joke; a cleaner intruding with a noisy floor polisher through the curtain around the bed where the body lay; the deaf patient in the next bed with the radio on maximum volume. It was as if the Devil was mocking us: *that's* your 'death with dignity'?

⌒

My office was in the same building at the back of the ministry where I had first stayed as a resident medical student in 1980. I was one of six; we were told to spend a week living on site, but, other than that, were given no guidance. We hung around the emergency department – then a small unit – but felt we were only getting in the way, so we spent most of the time watching TV in the doctors' lounge. One of our group was a tremendous show-off: he joshed and talked knowledgeably with the senior house officers and registrars. 'Have you taken that appendix to theatre yet?' he would ask, in his jaunty way.

The little galley kitchen where we made our coffee was around the corner from the office I now occupied. I could have sworn the cups we used in 1980 were still there. Sitting now, forty years on, in the same building, I thought about these cups, and dismissed them as a clunky, rather too obvious metaphor.

In the car park, the oncologist asked if it was true that I was retiring. A film buff, he warned me that one of the commonest movie plot lines was the ageing hero, just about to retire, when 'all hell breaks loose'. This would be my last night on call.

The Garden of Earthly Delights

It was a miserable morning, fog-bound and freezing, still dark when I arrived at 6.20. Just inside the main entrance of the ministry, a small crowd had gathered around a portable flimsy screen. Thinking someone had collapsed, I went to help. Three security men in high-visibility jackets were on the ground, restraining a young man who was thrashing and shouting. Another young man looked on.

The emergency department was a scene of horror, beyond the imaginings of Dickens or Hogarth; Florence Nightingale might have blanched – I can't imagine Scutari Hospital was any worse than this. Even the department's location – at the very rear of the original ministry building – suggested something *cloacal*. Years before, a very patrician doctor, shocked by a rare visit to the department, said, in a trembling voice: 'My God, it's like a scene from Hieronymus Bosch.' On this, my last visit, the emergency department did indeed resemble the right panel of the painter's triptych *The Garden of Earthly Delights*. The corridors were packed with patients on trolleys, so crowded that it was difficult to get past. I heard the shouting of the waking drunks and the shrieking of a delirious woman. As well as the usual odour of urine, I was overpowered by the unmistakable sweet-sickly stench of melaena, that black, tarry mixture of semi-digested blood and faeces that is the hallmark of a stomach bleed.

All twenty patients admitted under my care were in this department. The other six on-call services (cardiology, geriatrics, oncology, renal medicine, neurology, acute medicine) between them had taken *eleven*. A nervous senior house officer took me to the first patient, a woman she had diagnosed as a 'hypertensive emergency' (dangerously high blood pressure). 'Have you examined the optic fundi?'* I asked.

'No.'

It took some time to find an ophthalmoscope. I tried, in vain, to visualise the woman's optic fundi, but the artificial light was so bright her pupils were tiny, too small for me to see through to the retina.

An elderly man with a fracture just above his knee joint was lying on a trolley. The orthopaedic surgeons refused to take him, arguing that his treatment would be 'conservative', meaning that *they* would not operate to repair this break. The orthopaedic surgeon on call happened to pass by as I was looking at this man. I stopped him and asked him to take the patient; he paused, scowled, and walked away.

As I stood at one of the computer terminals on the nurses' station, looking at the rays of this man's shattered knee, a junior

---

* In severe hypertension, the retina (optic fundus) at the back of the eye is often swollen and bleeding.

emergency department doctor, without warning or apology, suddenly drew a tape – just missing my face – between me and the screen, marking out a do-not-pass line for her department's morning roll call of patients. The final indignity on the final round. If I had a sword, I would have laid it down.

⁓

I had lunch with a paediatrician. Although he wore a novelty Christmas jumper and a Santa hat, his mood was not festive. I asked if this jaunty seasonal apparel was obligatory on the children's ward. 'You get fined if you don't,' he confessed.

⁓

I went around the wards again in the afternoon. I went through every patient, every blood test, every X-ray. 'You must let the *chaps* [junior doctors] get on with it,' an NHS teaching hospital grandee advised me when I was promoted to consultant in the mid-1990s. 'The only way they learn is by doing it themselves.' One of the great delegators, he would be appalled by my micro-supervision of the *chaps*.

By 6 p.m., I had been in the hospital for nearly twelve hours and thought it might be safe to go home. As I left the office, my phone rang. It was Valerie, a former trainee, now a consultant in one of the rural hospitals. She had a man with liver disease whom she wanted to transfer.

'Valerie, I'd love to help, but there are no beds. All the patients I took last night are on trolleys in the emergency department.'

'I feel ashamed I can't look after him,' she said. 'I'm trained to do it, I know what to do, but I have no facilities here, no support. Nothing.'

I thought she was going to cry; only a year before, she had resigned from a good academic job in a Canadian teaching centre to come back to this little hospital, so strong was her desire to return to Ireland and raise her children here.

'I'll try to get him up after the weekend,' I promised, knowing this would be impossible. 'Happy Christmas, Valerie.'

'Last night was the first time I cried'

New year, new crisis. My colleagues, knowing that I would be retiring in February, had very generously relieved me of on-call and ward duties for my last Christmas. The ministry made the national TV news over the first weekend of the New Year with the highest number of patients on trolleys ever recorded. An emergency department nurse who had worked in the ministry for twelve years was interviewed on the main evening news. 'Last night was the first time I cried,' she said.

The nursing union demanded that all elective activity (which included my endoscopy list) be cancelled; the management acceded. Although cancellation of endoscopy day cases would not relieve in any way the trolley crisis – the endoscopy unit could not be reconfigured into an acute ward – the list was cancelled because both hospital management and the nursing union were desperate to convey an impression of decisive action.

My first outpatient of 2020 was a young woman with irritable bowel syndrome (IBS). Her IBS, she said, was 'manageable', but would I mind looking at her finger? She had injured it over the weekend. 'I didn't want to bother my GP, and I saw on TV how awful the emergency departments are.'

A man with worsening upper abdominal pain and vomiting was attending three clinics in two hospitals; no doctor had volunteered so far to be captain of this ship. I put him on the 'urgent' list for admission, not knowing when, or even if, this would happen.

A young man told me that he still had 'terrible pain from this anal fissure'. This discomfort was only surpassed by the cognitive dissonance he experienced when I told him that he did not have a fissure.

At the X-ray conference, I reviewed an ultrasound scan a GP had written to me about. She sent a patient for this scan to a private facility; they reported some tiny abnormality in the liver – almost certainly insignificant – but nevertheless recommended a CT scan. Since the patient did not have private insurance, the GP asked me to organise the scan. Tim reviewed the scan and pronounced it normal.

'Why don't you tell that GP to *fuck off*?' he suggested.

'I was tempted.'

'If I was retiring, I'd tell them all to fuck off.'

I wrote to the GP, advising her that a CT scan was not required. I did not, however, tell her to 'fuck off'.

⌒

I took a call from a bed manager asking if I still wanted them to transfer Valerie's patient.

'But I phoned you before Christmas about that man.'

'I know,' she said. 'It's been awful.'

I suggested that it might be best if I contacted Valerie again to find out what had happened over Christmas. I did. The man had died.

'Sorry, Valerie.'

'It's not your fault.'

⌒

When I was in my twenties, I wrote a play called *Ship of Fools*. The plot was very loosely based on the famous Rosenhan 'Thud' experiment. In 1973, David Rosenhan, a Stanford psychologist, published a paper in *Science* entitled 'On being sane in insane places'. He described how eight 'pseudopatients', who presented themselves to mental hospitals complaining that they heard voices saying 'hollow, empty and thud' – but no other 'symptoms' – were all immediately admitted, and seven of the eight were subsequently diagnosed as schizophrenic. The study caused a sensation at the time, questioning, as it did, the validity of psychiatric diagnosis and the long-term detainment of psychotic people. I came across a review of a new book, *The Great Pretender*, by Susannah Cahalan, which claims that much – probably most – of what Rosenhan wrote was fictitious; ironical, I suppose, given that his 'patients' presented with fictitious symptoms. These 'pseudopatients' were really *pseudopseudo*patients.

My play was never staged, a setback that I reacted to with all the stoicism and resilience of Bart Simpson, who when asked why he didn't keep up his guitar lessons, replied: 'I wasn't good at it right away, so I quit.'

For the next twenty-five years, any writing I did was technical, and published in specialist journals. And then I wrote about A. J. Cronin,* in a quixotic attempt to rescue him from neglect. My homage was published in one of those obscure quarterly journals produced by a royal college, but I felt a sense of accomplishment. An author whom I admired sent me an encouraging email. It was enough; I kept writing.

In my mid-fifties, I was overtaken by a compulsion to write about death, a common enough occurrence at the ministry, where 700 people died every year. This urge led to a book, in which I hinted at my medical apostasy. I made a full confession in my next book, *Can Medicine Be Cured?* This apostasy was now making my job increasingly untenable.

---

* A. J. Cronin was a Scottish doctor and novelist, a best-selling author from the 1930s to the 1960s. Dismissed as 'middlebrow', he is now largely forgotten. His most famous book, *The Citadel* (1937), is often credited as an influence on the foundation of the National Health Service in 1948.

'There was a brave doctor in Perth'

The receptionist at the outpatients whispered to me that the first patient at that day's clinic had been sent over from the adjacent adult mental health unit, where she was currently an inpatient. When I called her name, a small, elderly man emerged from the waiting room. 'I'd like to speak to you on my own first,' he said conspiratorially. I sat him down in the clinic room.

'We've met before,' he said.

'Have we?'

'I used to work in the dissecting room,' he smiled. I remembered. He was a technician in the anatomy department. He was kind to those students (like me) who were horrified by their first encounter with the pallid cadavers, the shock of cutting into that thick, waxy skin, through the marbled, butter-yellow subcutaneous fat.

'My heart is broken. My beautiful girl.' His forty-year-old daughter had been in the psychiatric unit for two months. Claire had been a brilliant student but was diagnosed with schizophrenia after a psychotic breakdown in her twenties; her life since then had been the usual tale of relapses, hospitalisations, medications. She had never worked and lived with her widowed father. 'What great hopes I had for her,' he said.

The psychiatrists sent her to me because they thought she had an abdominal mass; a CT scan showed cysts in her liver and kidneys. I invited Claire into the clinic room. She came in, shuffling along in her slippers* in short, Parkinsonian steps. She was forty but could have passed for sixty. Her abdomen was certainly protuberant, but there was no mass. I looked at the scans; the cysts were harmless. I reassured Claire and her father as best I could.

On the way out, he turned to his daughter, smiling: 'I knew him when he was a student. Now he's a *professor*.' I watched them as they left; the father stooped and old, the daughter so prematurely aged, she could have passed for his wife.

A woman complained of bad breath. 'I married the wrong man,' she sighed, 'and I have the neighbours from hell.' I sympathised, thinking I could do little about her poor choice of spouse or bad luck with neighbours, or indeed, her bad breath.

The GP's referral letter for the next patient contained this 'background' information: 'She became very stressed while on holiday in Thailand when she found out that her pension had been cut.'

---

* Why do patients with chronic psychosis nearly always wear slippers? The shuffle of slippers on polished floors is the defining sound of the psychiatric ward.

I continued the Augean task of clearing my office. It was like sorting through the personal effects of someone else, now dead, the random detritus of a career; much that once seemed important, journals that now I would never read. A research paper that was never published: I felt only relief. The trainee who had carried out (or perhaps *not* carried out) the experimental work for this so many years ago was, I suspected, a fraud. This suspicion took root only years later; I had no idea at the time. I fed the manuscript into the shredder, grateful that no journal had accepted it.

A letter, purporting to come from my outpatient clinic, forged by a patient addicted to opiates. So badly written, so clearly a fake; the 'letter' advised the GP to prescribe large doses of opiates, both orally and by injection, and concluded: 'we must now hope that the inflammation subsides', a sentence a doctor would *never* write.

A sheet of paper, given to me many years ago by a patient at the clinic. She wanted to make sure, she told me, that *everything* bothering her was listed. She described her symptoms in exquisitely beautiful handwriting – it was more like calligraphy; there were three perfectly executed drawings of her body, demonstrating the sites of pain. This work of art concluded: 'I would therefore be most grateful if you could find out what is wrong with me.'

*

Another sheet of paper, thin and yellow with age, given to me years before by a patient, an elderly man. He had written a poem in praise of the neurosurgical registrar who saved his life:

> There was a brave doctor in Perth
> Who was always on the alert
> A patient came in with life very slim
> He was thinking of leaving this earth.
>
> He complained of a violent pain in the head
> In a matter of minutes the man could be dead
> So with lightning decision he made an incision
> With a drill that he found in a shed.

He gave me several more poems; these included a tribute to Istabraq, the Irish horse who won the Champion Hurdle at Cheltenham in three successive years ('with fire in his belly and smoke out his arse'), and a celebration of Seamus Heaney's Nobel Prize:

> Here's a health to you Seamus Heaney
> You're the best we've ever seen
> Take a trip around Ireland
> In the state limousine.

The man on the phone

One of the acute physicians sent an email, suggesting a more equitable sharing of work in the division of medicine: 'An even distribution of the acute medical take among the stake-holding medical specialities avoids a rapid escalation of the inpatient census by respective teams on take.' A bit late for *me*, I thought.

⌒

A woman at the outpatients told me that her GP – whom I knew well – was 'red hot on diabetes'. This doctor viewed medicine primarily as a business. He had three surgeries, employing several salaried assistants. The key to success in general practice, he averred, was *turnover*: 'Get them out the fucking door within five minutes.' His 'turnover' was well into the millions, but since he had invested unwisely during the Celtic Tiger years – he had bought, as a member of a doctors' cartel, an entire shopping centre in Wales and an apartment building in Bulgaria, both of which crashed in value, losing most of the money invested – he would have to maintain this turnover indefinitely, and had to abandon his plan to retire to a Spanish golf resort. Despite this setback, his easy-going clubbable good humour was undented. He was always at the pint-drinking, back-slapping centre of any medical social event.

My next patient was a young woman with abdominal pain. Her notes documented a previous episode of leg weakness, which was given a label of 'dystonic posturing', a variant, according to her neurologist, of conversion disorder.*

A man with chronic diarrhoea told me that the only medication that worked for this was an acid-reducing medication called ranitidine. A branded version of this medication – which he believed to be the best – had been inexplicably taken off the market. I was about to tell him that this drug, the indications for which were heartburn, ulcers and gastritis, could not *possibly* ameliorate chronic diarrhoea, but thought: why bother? Why mess up his perfectly satisfactory arrangement with science, logic and evidence? I prescribed another acid-reducing medication (from the same family of drugs as ranitidine), reassuring him that this would be *just as effective* for his diarrhoea.

---

* Formerly known as 'hysterical conversion disorder,' the 'hysterical' bit was dropped after accusations of misogyny. Jean-Martin Charcot (1825–93), the famous French neurologist, used to display his hysterical patients like circus exhibits; many became famous in Paris for their 'performances'. Freud spent three months training with him and idolised *le professeur*: for the rest of his life he kept a bust of Charcot in his study.

*

A woman walked into the clinic room, pulling an oxygen cylinder on wheels; she had end-stage emphysema. She was worried, she said, about her bowels, oblivious of the lung disease that would kill her long before anything in her bowels would.

I lunched alone in the canteen, feeling an unexpected lightness. At the next table sat a man I had watched for years. He always ate alone; talking continuously on his phone, pausing only to consume a forkful of food. Whom did he talk to? Why did they never answer? Mid-forties; no uniform; he never smiled. He walked past, his phone cradled between shoulder and ear, and put his food tray on the conveyor belt.

A headline in *The Guardian*: 'Bed shortages leave Sunderland patients to sleep overnight in A&E'. This shortage had been going on for two decades in Ireland; sleeping overnight in A&E was *normal*.

A spokeswoman for the Irish health service was interviewed on radio yesterday and dismissed the number of people on trolleys as 'simply a manifestation of the very high turnover in our acute hospitals, and not in itself a cause for concern'.

The shredding company sent a lorry; they took away 3,000 sets of my private case notes and shredded them there and then in the lorry. I was invited to watch on video.

I had another vivid dream; this time, about a man whose cancer I missed at his first colonoscopy. He came back with further rectal bleeding a year later; I did another colonoscopy, finding a huge tumour. Dreams are always *true*: in dreams, you cannot lie, or rationalise, or make excuses. Freud was often right, but usually for the wrong reasons.

What would
Barry Marshall say?

A Moldovan man at the outpatients told me that his sore throat *and* headache had both been cured by a course of antibiotics given for *Helicobacter* infection. There was no plausible biological reason why this bacterium would cause either symptom. I silently invoked the spirits of the great statisticians, epidemiologists and prophets of evidence-based medicine, from Major Greenwood to Austin Bradford Hill to Archie Cochrane to David Sackett to John Ioannidis. Come, I said to them, come to my clinic and see for yourselves how little science matters! This is what my patients think of evidence!

The next patient must have read my thoughts. A woman with several complaints, including chronic cough, 'white phlegm', burping, bloating and chronic fatigue. She had a positive breath test for *Helicobacter* and was now convinced that all her woes were caused by this. I wondered what Barry Marshall* would say to this woman. 'I'm retiring' was a fabulously effective means of concluding a 'difficult' consultation.

I continued the office clear-out. A page I pulled from a magazine years ago, an interview with Bret Easton Ellis. Talking about depression and bereavement, he said that other people's sympathy was finite: 'In the end, your pain becomes a burden to them. Your pain is yours, not theirs.'

A collection of pencil drawings given to me by a patient who later died of cirrhosis. These were elaborate imaginary landscapes, childishly executed, full of castles, trees, swans, mountains. She whiled away her last days drawing these pictures. Although she was elderly and had been sick for a long time, on the day of her death her daughters were shocked, angry and somewhat hysterical. I recalled talking them down in the day room of the ward.

*

* The Australian gastroenterologist Barry Marshall shared the Nobel Prize in Medicine with Robin Warren (a pathologist) in 2005 for their discovery of the association of *Helicobacter* with gastritis and ulcers. Since this discovery, and particularly since the awarding of the Nobel Prize, *Helicobacter*-related duodenal ulcer – which once afflicted 10 per cent of the adult male population of Britain – has steadily declined. The main cause of gastric and duodenal ulcers now is non-steroidal anti-inflammatory drugs (including aspirin).

The *British Medical Journal* obituary of a friend who had killed herself. She was a musician; like William Carlos Williams, she grappled with the problem of *sustenance*, and switched from music to medicine. I think she paid for this decision with her life, consumed on the flaming ramparts of the world.

A copy of a long letter I wrote to a grieving family, a rare example of this being more truthful, and more informative (for *them*), than any conversation. Their mother had died under my care, the culmination of a three-year period when she had been admitted on sixteen occasions under eight consultants. The problem was not negligence or error, but the failure of any doctor to take charge, to be the captain of that ship. Neither patient nor family knew that her combination of chronic diseases would kill her, and sooner, not later. No one (including me) had bothered to take the time to have the difficult conversation, and her death came as a shock to her family. A meeting some weeks later ended acrimoniously. When the emotion had subsided, I sat down with the case notes, went through every detail of this woman's care, and wrote a long letter to her son. I was surprised and moved when he replied, thanking me for being honest and giving some peace of mind to the family: 'No one told us how sick she really was.'

The 'surprise' question: would you be *surprised* if this patient died within the next year? If the answer is 'no', we should automatically have the difficult conversation – no, the *essential* conversation. What misery we might spare our patients and their families. But we keep avoiding the surprise question; we go on pretending, *processing*.

*

I found old correspondence with hospital managers and clinical directors about being available out of hours when not officially on call. I read it with weariness, the anger now long spent. I thought of the dozens of phone calls that began: 'I know you're not on call but...' My children, long exposed to such unwelcome interruptions, had very early vowed not to follow me into medicine.

I shredded these ancient, mean-spirited letters.

The minutes of meetings of a pan-European committee I had once sat on, when I was an ambitious young careerist. This group concerned itself with 'quality' in endoscopy and was funded by the endoscope manufacturers. The members conformed to their national stereotypes: the Italians were Machiavellian schemers, permanently on their phones; the Germans methodical and humourless; the English blandly superior: 'You must remember, Jean-François...' We engaged in interminable specious debates on the correct terminology to describe abnormalities (such as ulcers) detected by endoscopy.

The last meeting of this committee I attended was held in a grey concrete airport hotel in Amsterdam; on the flight home, I promised myself I would never go back. I dropped out of the threepenny handicap race for academic promotion and went my own way. I would never again have to feign interest in the semiotics of endoscopy.

*

A handwritten, laminated copy of the oath of Maimonides* given to me many years ago by a patient, a Dublin-born Jewish woman who lived in Leeds:

... may neither avarice nor miserliness, nor thirst for glory or for a great reputation engage my mind...

May I never see in the patient anything but a fellow creature in pain.

---

* Maimonides (1138–1204) was a Sephardic Jewish physician, philosopher and astronomer. (*Probably* a polymath.) This oath, although attributed to Maimonides, was almost certainly written by the German-Jewish physician Markus Herz in 1793.

'Could it be nerves?'

The grand round was given by a trainee anaesthetist, a young man of thirty, who talked about the climate crisis. With his beard, blue scrubs top and mid-Atlantic accent, I wanted to dislike him, but he was entirely convincing. He mocked climate sceptics with a slide called: 'What if it's a big hoax and we created a better world for nothing?'

⤿

My last outpatient clinic. Two people with 'medically unexplained symptoms' expressed frustration with their normal test results. One communicated this disappointment through a Polish interpreter.

'Could it be nerves?' asked the second; at last, I thought, a *breakthrough*.

'Yes, it *could*,' I said, gently encouraging this new psychological narrative.

She pointed at her belly. 'Which nerve?'

*

A man in his late sixties told me that he had once spent a year in bed with fatigue; he attributed this to an antifungal drug he had taken for athlete's foot. Now, he told me, he woke several times a night.

'Why?'

'To massage the stool around my colon.'

A man sent by his GP with episodes of choking.

'When did you last have this?' I asked.

'Two years ago,' he replied, somewhat sheepishly. 'I told my GP I was fine, but she insisted I keep this appointment.'

On it went, somehow, this sclerotic system; the GPs kept referring this stuff, like pouring water into a blocked drain and looking away.

A jolly man of seventy, referred by his GP for investigation of his chronic burping. The upper lobe of his right lung had been removed four years earlier for cancer; he had never smoked. The diagnosis was fortuitous; he was knocked over by a cow and went to hospital with broken ribs. The chest X-ray revealed not only several cracked ribs, but also a cancer, small enough to be cured. 'The cow is sacred,' he laughed.

A morbidly obese, homeless Romanian woman sent by the cardiologists for investigation of mild anaemia, probably due to aspirin. She had multiple conditions, including diabetes, emphysema and heart disease. This anaemia was trifling, the least of her worries, but here she was, at my clinic, and would have to be booked for investigations. How do you prepare a homeless diabetic for colonoscopy? She would have to be brought in, but with the bed situation being what it was, that could take months.

The communication skills experts taught the medical students, when taking a history, to let the patient speak, without interruption, until they had finished their story.* This strategy (or was it a tactic?) was of little use in the overcrowded clinics where I had spent my career. My final patient, a woman in her forties, spoke for ten minutes; I did not interrupt her. Just when I thought she had reached the conclusion ('those are the issues, I suppose'), off she would go again. No detail was too negligible. I wrote down *everything* she said, as if she was my very first, not my last ever patient.

I attended the funeral mass of a classmate, the surgeon who died after the now obligatory 'long battle' with cancer. People often say 'I was humbled' when they have been given an award or a prize, or in some way elevated or recognised, when they felt anything but 'humbled'. But 'humbled' was the right word

---

* Wilfred Trotter, wrote Julian Taylor, listened 'attentively to the longest and most rambling story alike from the neurote and the husky old slum lady, with the same courtesy that he probably paid to duchesses... He never interrupted.'

today. His wife was not there to mourn him; although only in her mid-sixties, she was now in a nursing home. His five children, all grown now, were heartbroken but proud. He lived with both the cancer and his wife's decline for more than five years. I do not suppose that he lay awake at night cursing this fate. I think he embraced it: *amor fati*. He was equal to it.

The church was packed; I recognised many doctors. One, sitting in my pew, untroubled by the proximity of a dead colleague in a coffin, complained loudly about his plantar fasciitis,* and how it limited his golf and skiing. Two sworn enemies shook hands; their *ad hominem* correspondence, conducted when, years before, they were chairs of their respective divisions, and copied to all the doctors in these divisions, was unintentionally hilarious, full of hysterical contempt.

After mass I sheltered from the icy rain with a group of classmates in the church porch. When it cleared, we went for coffee. An old friend, long settled in London, where he was now a professor, was disapproving when I told him I would soon retire. '*I* wouldn't dream of going so early!' he said, and then admitted that he had offloaded his on-call commitment. Another classmate, a GP, told me about the methadone clinic he ran. 'They're entitled to free dental care,' he said. 'They all have gleaming new implants.'

---

* Plantar fasciitis is an inflammatory disorder of the fibrous tissue (plantar fascia) along the sole of the foot. It typically causes stabbing pain in the heel.

'What's the story with this virus?'

My last day as a doctor. I rose early and was at my desk by eight. A letter from the hospice, informing me of the death of a patient with a rare form of cancer, admitted there after 'entering a phase of accelerated decline'. The palliative care consultant wrote: 'The patient demonstrated limited insight into the nature of his disease.' Another C-minus. My patients will really have to do better at dying.

⌣

A knock on my door. It was Helen, a clerical officer, with a card for me and a box of Jacob's USA biscuits.

⌣

Dominic, the endoscopy receptionist, shook his head, ruefully, theatrically. 'We lost at home *again*.' His main concern – and only topic of conversation – was the fortunes of Leeds United. The club's long banishment from the Premier League was, for Dominic, a source of perpetual sorrow, as well as mockery from his workmates who supported more successful teams. Dominic was a boy when Leeds dominated English football, and his heroes were John Giles, Billy Bremner and Norman Hunter. It had been a tough fifteen years since relegation in 2004, the nadir reached when the club dropped to the depths of the third tier of English football in 2007. I would often talk with Dominic about Leeds; he was impressed by the fact that I had lived in the city for nearly ten years, and was an occasional visitor to the club's ground, Elland Road. When the endoscopy nurses interrupted these conversations to ask him to clerk in a patient, Dominic would look at them with his big brown eyes, like a figure from the foot of an El Greco crucifixion, and beseech them: 'Don't you know I've only one pair of hands?'

The last patient for colonoscopy on the list – now the last of my *career* – had a huge tumour.

The endoscopy nurses gave me tea and cake; a colleague gave a short, graceful speech.

⌒

During my sparsely attended last tutorial on 'Literature and Medicine', I somehow strayed on to the 'trolley crisis'.

'Are we ever going to *fix* this?' a young man asked.

'My generation failed. Over to you.'

Walking out the back entrance by the emergency department, I met Little Tommy's dad.

'Tommy's dead.'

He had collapsed at home. He was rushed by ambulance to the resus room; they worked on Little Tommy for an hour before calling 'time'.

'You knew him,' he said.

On the way to my office, I met my friend Con, the microbiologist; he was not in good humour, having just emerged from a meeting about coronavirus.

'What's the story with this virus?' I asked.

'Fuck knows.'

Towards the end of the 1972 film *Jeremiah Johnson*, Johnson (Robert Redford) meets his old mentor, the trapper called Bear Claw (Will Geer). Since their last meeting, Johnson has endured the most appalling violence and hardship.

'You've come far, pilgrim,' says Bear Claw.

'Feels like far,' replies Johnson.

'Were it worth the trouble?'

'Huh? What trouble?'

I felt a tenderness for my younger self: I could not have known better or done it differently. The multiple potential permutations of my lost and irretrievable past were as chaff. There was no parallel universe where I didn't make those mistakes, where I was a better, kinder, wiser person. I am as I am, the world is as it is. It was the best job in the world; it was the worst job in the world. Lurching between boredom and terror, no other career gave you so many opportunities to fail.

It was cold, wet, and windy. I handed back my office key and staff card, loaded the last of my possessions into the car boot, and drove home. I had survived, but was *survival* enough?

Epilogue

I retired on 7 February 2020, the day before my sixtieth birthday. A friend asked how I felt about it.

'It's just a job, like any other,' I said glibly.

'No, it's not,' he replied.

He was right.

On 11 February, the WHO named the new disease 'COVID-19'. In mid-March, I volunteered to return to clinical duties. I was not called. The weekly wellbeing messages mysteriously stopped. Leeds United were finally promoted.

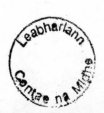

Acknowledgements

Acknowledgements

My editor Neil Belton first suggested the subject, and shepherded this book through several versions. I am very grateful to him, and to his colleague Clare Gordon for their unwavering support. Jenni Davis's copy-editing was meticulous. Thanks also to my agent Jonathan Williams. My brother David has long championed Mr Wolfe as a model of efficiency and grace under pressure. I am grateful to Paul Mulholland, editor of the *Medical Independent*, where I have written about some of the themes of this book.